MW01241097

A Gift For:

....

From:

....

C·R·E·A·T·I·O·N Health

ONE
SENTENCE
JOURNAL
a three-year record

Todd Chobotar

General Editor

creation
HEALTH

To Extend *the* Healing Ministry *of* Christ

General Editor:	Todd Chobotar
Production:	Lillian Boyd
Copy Editor:	Mollie Braga
Cover Design:	Carter Design
Interior Design:	Timothy Brown

Publisher's Note: This book is not intended to replace a one-on-one relationship with a qualified healthcare professional. You are advised and encouraged to consult with your healthcare professional in all matters relating to your health and the health of your family. The publisher disclaims any liability arising directly or indirectly from the use of this book.

Unless otherwise noted, all Scripture quotations are from the *Holy Bible, New Living Translation*, Copyright © 1996, 2004, 2007, 2013 by Tyndale House Publishers, Inc., Carol Stream, IL 60188. Other Scripture references are from the following sources: *The Living Bible* (TLB) copyright © 1971, by Tyndale House Publishers, Inc., Carol Stream, IL 60188. *Common English Bible®* (CEB) copyright © 2010, 2011 by Common English Bible™. *Good News Translation* (GNT) copyright © 1992 by American Bible Society. *New King James Version* (NKJV) Copyright © 1979, 1982 by Thomas Nelson. *The Holy Bible, New International Version* (NIV) copyright © 1973, 1978, 1984, 2011 by Biblica, Inc.™ Used by permission of Zondervan. All translations used by permission. All rights reserved worldwide.

For volume discounts please contact special sales at:
HealthProducts@FLHosp.org | 407-303-1929

ISBN 13: 978-0-9887406-0-0

For other life changing resources visit:
FloridaHospitalPublishing.com
CREATIONHealth.com

WELCOME

What is **CREATION** Health?

CREATION Health is a holistic lifestyle program for those who want to live healthier, happier lives. The eight wellness principles of CREATION Health are: Choice, Rest, Environment, Activity, Trust, Interpersonal Relationships, Outlook, and Nutrition. You'll find a short summary for each of these principles at the bottom of the journaling pages ahead. These principles have a long, proven history of promoting greater health and longevity worldwide.

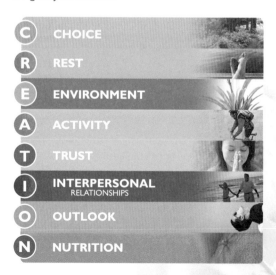

C CHOICE

R REST

E ENVIRONMENT

A ACTIVITY

T TRUST

I INTERPERSONAL
RELATIONSHIPS

O OUTLOOK

N NUTRITION

What is a One-Sentence Journal?

A One-Sentence Journal is a simple, fun way to
record your day-to-day life. It's a dedicated space
where you take a few moments (usually at the end
of your day) to pause, reflect, and record what
transpired or inspired you today.

Why only one sentence? Well, most of us are busy
people. Perhaps you've tried to keep a journal
before, but gave up because it took too much time,
or you were too tired to write long entries. If so, the
One-Sentence Journal is perfect for you. It's a little
bit of time that adds up to big life change.

How Will I Benefit From Using This Journal?

Journaling has many benefits.

First, journaling helps you grow as a person. It helps
identify your goals and values. It can clarify your
behaviors and demonstrate your life's potential.
It causes you to be less reactive and more reflective.
It gives your mind a mental workout. Journaling can
bring focus to your day and teach you more about
how you process the world around you.

Second, journaling can reduce stress and bring healing into your life. It gives you a place to express honest emotions that you might be hesitant to share elsewhere. It can untangle thoughts and feelings. It may assist you in releasing pain from your past and opening a new door to freedom. Journaling empowers you to take greater control of your life. Many people report that journaling helps them understand more about themselves, their relationships, and their life circumstances.

Third, journaling enhances your creativity. It makes you look at the world in a different way—sometimes offering new perspectives you hadn't considered before. It can bring about new ideas or insights. It teaches you how to write your story and the stories of those you love. Journaling is a form of self-expression that can lead to creative breakthroughs.

Finally, journaling helps you recall the past and revitalize the present. It aids you in tracking life's most important moments. It can help you remember both the valleys and mountaintops of life. It can help you spot patterns you might not have otherwise noticed. Journaling can awaken a sense of gratitude and help you feel more spiritually connected.

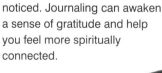

How Should I Use This One-Sentence Journal?

Need some ideas for what to write about? No problem. Turn to the inside back cover. There's a whole list of ideas. A kind of Quick Reference Guide of topics to spur your imagination!

When you write, use variety. Try different ideas and topics. It helps keep you interested. Most importantly, *have fun!* Let your One-Sentence Journal reflect who you are as a person.

By the way, ***don't wait*** to start journaling till January 1. Simply turn to today's date and begin. When you finish the year, start the next. In your second and third year, be sure to read your previous entries from that day. It's a great way to recall the past and inspire you in the present.

Okay, you're ready to go. Enjoy!

Here's to your good health,

Todd Chobotar
General Editor

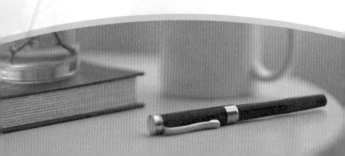

JANUARY 1

*Choice is a power and a privilege our heavenly Father
has given all of us. What will you do with yours?*
Delores Francois

20__: _____

_____

_____

_____

20__: _____

_____

_____

_____

20__: _____

_____

_____

_____

CHOICE – First we make choices,
then choices make us. Choose an
inspiring destination, then create a set
of healthy habits to get you there.

JANUARY 2

. . . .

*By tapping into the power of the Spirit, you can
take Jesus' yoke upon you, learn from him,
and find rest for your soul.*
Dr. Dick Tibbits

20__: _____

_____

_____

_____

20__: _____

_____

_____

_____

20__: _____

_____

_____

_____

REST – Rest rebuilds the mind, body,
and spirit. The best rest includes a
sanctuary of time set aside to rejuvenate
daily, weekly, and annually.

JANUARY 3

....

*A man's character always takes its hue, more or less,
from the form and color of things about him.*
Frederick Douglass

20__: _____

_____

_____

_____

20__: _____

_____

_____

_____

20__: _____

_____

_____

_____

E **ENVIRONMENT** – All of your
senses—sight, smell, sound, touch, and
taste—influence your mood and your
health. So optimize your environment.

JANUARY 4

To enjoy the glow of good health, you must exercise.
Gene Tunney

20__: _____

_____

_____

_____

20__: _____

_____

_____

_____

20__: _____

_____

_____

_____

ACTIVITY – Activity includes both mental and physical strengthening. A fit mind promotes a healthy body, and a healthy body promotes a fit mind.

JANUARY 5

....

Blessed is the one who trusts in the Lord,
whose confidence is in him.
Jeremiah 17:7 (NIV)

20__: _____

_____

_____

_____

20__: _____

_____

_____

_____

20__: _____

_____

_____

_____

TRUST – Trust in God can promote
better health. Faith, hope, and love
provide lasting peace and may help you
live a longer, happier life.

JANUARY 6

Things are never quite as scary when you've got a best friend.
Bill Watterson

20__: _____

_____

_____

_____

20__: _____

_____

_____

_____

20__: _____

_____

_____

_____

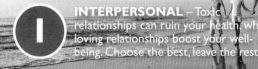

I **INTERPERSONAL** – Toxic relationships can ruin your health, while loving relationships boost your well-being. Choose the best, leave the rest.

JANUARY 7

....

Failure is simply the opportunity to begin again more intelligently.
Henry Ford

20__: _____

_____

_____

_____

20__: _____

_____

_____

_____

20__: _____

_____

_____

_____

 OUTLOOK – Attitude influences outcome. Your outlook can impact the progression of disease or the increase of health. Choose to stay positive today.

JANUARY 8

....

With all the concerns about diet today, here's the
real bottom line: keep it simple.
Des Cummings Jr., PhD

20__: _____
_____
_____
_____

20__: _____
_____
_____
_____

20__: _____
_____
_____
_____

NUTRITION – Food is the fuel that
drives your life. It can rev you up or slow
you down. Evaluate your intake. Eat for
energy. Eat for life!

JANUARY 9

. . . .

The strongest principle of growth lies in the human choice.
George Elliot

20__: _____

_____

_____

_____

20__: _____

_____

_____

_____

20__: _____

_____

_____

_____

CHOICE – First we make choices, then choices make us. Choose an inspiring destination, then create a set of healthy habits to get you there.

JANUARY 10

*The week's end was designed to enable us to release the mental
load of the workweek and reconnect with those relationships
we value most—our families, our friends, ourselves, our God.*

Monica Reed, MD

20__: _____

_____

_____

_____

20__: _____

_____

_____

_____

20__: _____

_____

_____

_____

REST – Rest rebuilds the mind, body,
and spirit. The best rest includes a
sanctuary of time set aside to rejuvenate
daily, weekly, and annually.

JANUARY 11

*I think you might dispense with half your doctors
if you would only consult Dr. Sun more.*
Henry Ward Beecher

20__: _____

_____

_____

_____

20__: _____

_____

_____

_____

20__: _____

_____

_____

_____

E **ENVIRONMENT** – All of your
senses—sight, smell, sound, touch, and
taste—influence your mood and your
health. So optimize your environment.

JANUARY 12

Yesterday you said tomorrow. Just do it.
Nike

20__ : _____

_____

_____

_____

20__ : _____

_____

_____

_____

20__ : _____

_____

_____

_____

ACTIVITY – Activity includes both mental and physical strengthening. A fit mind promotes a healthy body, and a healthy body promotes a fit mind.

JANUARY 13

If life gets too hard to stand, kneel.
Gordon B. Hinckley

20__: _____

_____

_____

_____

20__: _____

_____

_____

_____

20__: _____

_____

_____

_____

TRUST – Trust in God can promote better health. Faith, hope, and love provide lasting peace and may help you live a longer, happier life.

JANUARY 14

. . . .

The meeting of two personalities is like the contact of two
chemical substances: if there is any reaction,
both are transformed.
C.G. Jung

20__: _____

_____

_____

_____

20__: _____

_____

_____

_____

20__: _____

_____

_____

_____

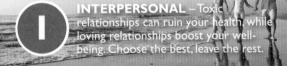

INTERPERSONAL – Toxic
relationships can ruin your health, while
loving relationships boost your well-
being. Choose the best, leave the rest.

JANUARY 15

. . . .

OPPORTUNITYISNOWHERE. Do you see "opportunity is now here" or "opportunity is nowhere"?
Lynell LaMountain

20__: _____

_____

_____

_____

20__: _____

_____

_____

_____

20__: _____

_____

_____

_____

OUTLOOK – Attitude influences outcome. Your outlook can impact the progression of disease or the increase of health. Choose to stay positive today.

JANUARY 16

Water is the only drink of a wise man.
Henry David Thoreau

20__: _____

_____

_____

_____

20__: _____

_____

_____

_____

20__: _____

_____

_____

_____

NUTRITION – Food is the fuel that
drives your life. It can rev you up or slow
you down. Evaluate your intake. Eat for
energy. Eat for life!

JANUARY 17

. . . .

I, not events, have the power to make me happy or unhappy today.
I can choose which it shall be. Yesterday is dead, tomorrow
hasn't arrived yet. I have just one day, today, and I'm
going to be happy in it.   Groucho Marx

20__: _____

_____

_____

_____

20__: _____

_____

_____

_____

20__: _____

_____

_____

_____

CHOICE – First we make choices,
then choices make us. Choose an
inspiring destination, then create a set
of healthy habits to get you there.

JANUARY 18

*A day out-of-doors, someone I loved to talk with,
a good book and some simple food and
music—that would be rest.*
Eleanor Roosevelt

20__: _____

_____

_____

_____

20__: _____

_____

_____

_____

20__: _____

_____

_____

_____

REST – Rest rebuilds the mind, body,
and spirit. The best rest includes a
sanctuary of time set aside to rejuvenate
daily, weekly, and annually.

JANUARY 19

Simplicity is the ultimate sophistication.
Leonardo Da Vinci

20__: _____

_____

_____

_____

20__: _____

_____

_____

_____

20__: _____

_____

_____

_____

ENVIRONMENT – All of your senses—sight, smell, sound, touch, and taste—influence your mood and your health. So optimize your environment.

JANUARY 20

*A vigorous five-mile walk will do more good for an unhappy
but otherwise healthy adult than all the medicine
and psychology in the world.*
Paul Dudley White

20__: _____

_____

_____

_____

20__: _____

_____

_____

_____

20__: _____

_____

_____

_____

ACTIVITY – Activity includes both
mental and physical strengthening. A fit
mind promotes a healthy body, and a
healthy body promotes a fit mind.

JANUARY 21

. . . .

*Today, I don't claim to know very much, but I know I have a greater
scope and a broader perspective because of the intimacy I
have been given with the One who does know all things.*
Linda Nordyke Hambleton

20___: _____

_____

_____

_____

20___: _____

_____

_____

_____

20___: _____

_____

_____

_____

TRUST – Trust in God can promote
better health. Faith, hope, and love
provide lasting peace and may help you
live a longer, happier life.

JANUARY 22

A successful marriage requires falling in love many times, always with the same person.
Mignon McLaughlin

20__: _____

_____

_____

_____

20__: _____

_____

_____

_____

20__: _____

_____

_____

_____

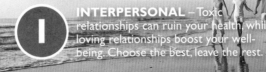

INTERPERSONAL – Toxic relationships can ruin your health, while loving relationships boost your well-being. Choose the best, leave the rest.

JANUARY 23

. . . .

You see, over time, your outer world becomes
a reflection of your inner world.
Dr. Dick Tibbits

20__: _____

_____

_____

_____

20__: _____

_____

_____

_____

20__: _____

_____

_____

_____

OUTLOOK – Attitude influences
outcome. Your outlook can impact the
progression of disease or the increase of
health. Choose to stay positive today.

JANUARY 24

. . . .

"Breaking bread" together deepens relationships
and nourishes our souls.
Monica Reed, MD

20__: _____

_____

_____

_____

20__: _____

_____

_____

_____

20__: _____

_____

_____

_____

NUTRITION – Food is the fuel that
drives your life. It can rev you up or slow
you down. Evaluate your intake. Eat for
energy. Eat for life!

JANUARY 25

....

But if serving the Lord seems undesirable to you, then choose for
yourselves this day whom you will serve ... But as for me
and my household, we will serve the Lord.
Joshua 24:15 (NIV)

20__: _____

_____

_____

_____

20__: _____

_____

_____

_____

20__: _____

_____

_____

_____

CHOICE – First we make choices,
then choices make us. Choose an
inspiring destination, then create a set
of healthy habits to get you there.

JANUARY 26

*Slow down and everything you are chasing
will come around and catch you.*
John De Paola

20__: _____

_____

_____

_____

20__: _____

_____

_____

_____

20__: _____

_____

_____

_____

REST – Rest rebuilds the mind, body,
and spirit. The best rest includes a
sanctuary of time set aside to rejuvenate
daily, weekly, and annually.

JANUARY 27

. . . .

The best place to find God is in a garden.
You can dig for him there.
George Bernard Shaw

20__: _____

_____

_____

_____

20__: _____

_____

_____

_____

20__: _____

_____

_____

_____

E

ENVIRONMENT – All of your
senses—sight, smell, sound, touch, and
taste—influence your mood and your
health. So optimize your environment.

JANUARY 28

. . . .

If you don't feel as though you have the time to exercise,
then take a good long look at your schedule
and see what you can cut out....
Sherri Flynt, MPH, RD, LD

20__: _____

_____

_____

_____

20__: _____

_____

_____

_____

20__: _____

_____

_____

_____

ACTIVITY – Activity includes both mental and physical strengthening. A fit mind promotes a healthy body, and a healthy body promotes a fit mind.

JANUARY 29

Faith in God includes faith in his timing.
Neal A. Maxwell

20__: _____

_____

_____

_____

20__: _____

_____

_____

_____

20__: _____

_____

_____

_____

TRUST – Trust in God can promote better health. Faith, hope, and love provide lasting peace and may help you live a longer, happier life.

JANUARY 30

....

The missing ingredient in many unhappy
marriages isn't love, but friendship.
Todd Chobotar

20__: _____

_____

_____

_____

20__: _____

_____

_____

_____

20__: _____

_____

_____

_____

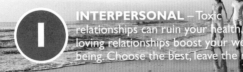

I

INTERPERSONAL – Toxic
relationships can ruin your health, while
loving relationships boost your well-
being. Choose the best, leave the rest.

JANUARY 31

....

Hope is the most powerful stimulant for the body.
John Harvey Kellogg, MD

20__: _____

_____

_____

_____

20__: _____

_____

_____

_____

20__: _____

_____

_____

_____

OUTLOOK – Attitude influences
outcome. Your outlook can impact the
progression of disease or the increase of
health. Choose to stay positive today.

FEBRUARY 1

*So whether you eat or drink or whatever
you do, do it all for the glory of God.*
1 Corinthians 10:31

20__: _____

_____

_____

20__: _____

_____

_____

20__: _____

_____

_____

_____

NUTRITION – Food is the fuel that
drives your life. It can rev you up or slow
you down. Evaluate your intake. Eat for
energy. Eat for life!

FEBRUARY 2

. . . .

It is easier to prevent bad habits than to break them.
Benjamin Franklin

20__: _____

_____

_____

_____

20__: _____

_____

_____

_____

20__: _____

_____

_____

_____

CHOICE – First we make choices, then choices make us. Choose an inspiring destination, then create a set of healthy habits to get you there.

FEBRUARY 3

*Praise be to the Lord, who has given rest to his
people Israel just as he promised.*
1 Kings 8:56 (NIV)

20__: _____

_____

_____

_____

20__: _____

_____

_____

_____

20__: _____

_____

_____

_____

REST – Rest rebuilds the mind, body,
and spirit. The best rest includes a
sanctuary of time set aside to rejuvenate
daily, weekly, and annually.

FEBRUARY 4

*Imagine sitting quietly in the middle of God's garden with only the
sounds of nature filling your ears and calming your spirit: birds
chirping, a brook flowing, the breeze gently rustling leaves.*
Des Cummings Jr., PhD

20__: _____

_____

_____

_____

20__: _____

_____

_____

_____

20__: _____

_____

_____

_____

E **ENVIRONMENT** – All of your
senses—sight, smell, sound, touch, and
taste—influence your mood and your
health. So optimize your environment.

FEBRUARY 5

Sweat is weakness leaving the body.
ADIDAS

20___: _____

_____

_____

_____

20___: _____

_____

_____

_____

20___: _____

_____

_____

_____

ACTIVITY – Activity includes both mental and physical strengthening. A fit mind promotes a healthy body, and a healthy body promotes a fit mind.

FEBRUARY 6

*I have been driven many times to my knees by the overwhelming
conviction that I had nowhere to go. My own wisdom, and
that of all about me, seemed insufficient for the day.*
Abraham Lincoln

20__: _____

_____

_____

_____

20__: _____

_____

_____

_____

20__: _____

_____

_____

_____

TRUST – Trust in God can promote
better health. Faith, hope, and love
provide lasting peace and may help you
live a longer, happier life.

FEBRUARY 7

Above all, love each other deeply, because
love covers over a multitude of sins.
I Peter 4:8 (NIV)

20__: _____

_____

_____

_____

20__: _____

_____

_____

_____

20__: _____

_____

_____

_____

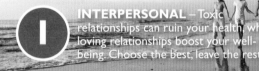

I **INTERPERSONAL** – Toxic
relationships can ruin your health, while
loving relationships boost your well-
being. Choose the best, leave the rest.

FEBRUARY 8

. . . .

Your positive mental outlook begins the moment you
determine to make the most of any situation
in which you find yourself.
Monica Reed, MD

20__: _____

_____

_____

_____

20__: _____

_____

_____

_____

20__: _____

_____

_____

_____

OUTLOOK – Attitude influences
outcome. Your outlook can impact the
progression of disease or the increase of
health. Choose to stay positive today.

FEBRUARY 9

*The food you eat can either be the safest and
most powerful form of medicine or the
slowest form of poison.*
Ann Wigmore

20__: _____

_____

_____

_____

20__: _____

_____

_____

_____

20__: _____

_____

_____

_____

NUTRITION – Food is the fuel that
drives your life. It can rev you up or slow
you down. Evaluate your intake. Eat for
energy. Eat for life!

FEBRUARY 10

What is right is often forgotten by what is convenient.
Bodie Thoene

20__: _____

_____

_____

_____

20__: _____

_____

_____

_____

20__: _____

_____

_____

_____

CHOICE – First we make choices, then choices make us. Choose an inspiring destination, then create a set of healthy habits to get you there.

FEBRUARY 11

Let's begin by taking a smallish nap or two....
A.A. Milne

20__: _____

_____

_____

_____

20__: _____

_____

_____

_____

20__: _____

_____

_____

_____

REST – Rest rebuilds the mind, body, and spirit. The best rest includes a sanctuary of time set aside to rejuvenate daily, weekly, and annually.

FEBRUARY 12

....

The best remedy for those who are afraid, lonely, or unhappy
is to go outside, somewhere where they can be quite
alone with the heavens, nature, and God.
Anne Frank

20__: _____

_____

_____

_____

20__: _____

_____

_____

_____

20__: _____

_____

_____

_____

E

ENVIRONMENT – All of your
senses—sight, smell, sound, touch, and
taste—influence your mood and your
health. So optimize your environment.

FEBRUARY 13

Happiness is a state of activity.
Aristotle

20__: _____

_____

_____

_____

20__: _____

_____

_____

_____

20__: _____

_____

_____

_____

ACTIVITY – Activity includes both mental and physical strengthening. A fit mind promotes a healthy body, and a healthy body promotes a fit mind.

FEBRUARY 14

Prayer is talk—honest talk, fearless talk, friend to friend.
Des Cummings Jr., PhD

20__: _____

_____

_____

20__: _____

_____

_____

20__: _____

_____

_____

_____

TRUST – Trust in God can promote better health. Faith, hope, and love provide lasting peace and may help you live a longer, happier life.

FEBRUARY 15

. . . .

Flee the evil desires of youth and pursue righteousness,
faith, love and peace, along with those who
call on the Lord out of a pure heart.
2 Timothy 2:22 (NIV)

20__: _____

_____

_____

_____

20__: _____

_____

_____

_____

20__: _____

_____

_____

_____

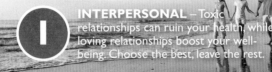

I **INTERPERSONAL** – Toxic relationships can ruin your health, while loving relationships boost your well-being. Choose the best, leave the rest.

FEBRUARY 16

. . . .

*Most people are about as happy as they
make up their minds to be.*
Abraham Lincoln

20__: _____

_____

_____

_____

20__: _____

_____

_____

_____

_____

20__: _____

_____

_____

_____

_____

OUTLOOK – Attitude influences
outcome. Your outlook can impact the
progression of disease or the increase of
health. Choose to stay positive today.

FEBRUARY 17

People who love to eat are always the best people.
Julia Child

20__: _____

_____

_____

_____

20__: _____

_____

_____

_____

20__: _____

_____

_____

_____

NUTRITION – Food is the fuel that drives your life. It can rev you up or slow you down. Evaluate your intake. Eat for energy. Eat for life!

FEBRUARY 18

*There are two primary choices in life: to accept
conditions as they exist, or accept the
responsibility for changing them.*
Denis Waitley

20__: _____

_____

_____

_____

20__: _____

_____

_____

_____

20__: _____

_____

_____

_____

CHOICE – First we make choices,
then choices make us. Choose an
inspiring destination, then create a set
of healthy habits to get you there.

FEBRUARY 19

Napping is a tool as old as time itself.
A. Roger Ekirch

20__: _____

_____

_____

_____

20__: _____

_____

_____

_____

20__: _____

_____

_____

_____

REST – Rest rebuilds the mind, body, and spirit. The best rest includes a sanctuary of time set aside to rejuvenate daily, weekly, and annually.

FEBRUARY 20

Every minute outside and awake is a good minute.
Bill Watterson

20__: _____

_____

_____

_____

20__: _____

_____

_____

_____

20__: _____

_____

_____

_____

ENVIRONMENT – All of your senses—sight, smell, sound, touch, and taste—influence your mood and your health. So optimize your environment.

FEBRUARY 21

Being active is not a matter of appearance, fashion, or form.
Art Bakewell

20__: _____

_____

_____

_____

20__: _____

_____

_____

_____

20__: _____

_____

_____

_____

ACTIVITY – Activity includes both mental and physical strengthening. A fit mind promotes a healthy body, and a healthy body promotes a fit mind.

FEBRUARY 22

*To be a Christian means to forgive the inexcusable because
God has forgiven the inexcusable in you.*
C.S. Lewis

20__: _____

_____

_____

_____

20__: _____

_____

_____

_____

20__: _____

_____

_____

_____

TRUST – Trust in God can promote
better health. Faith, hope, and love
provide lasting peace and may help you
live a longer, happier life.

FEBRUARY 23

How lucky I am to have something that
makes saying goodbye so hard.
A.A. Milne

20__: _____

_____

_____

_____

20__: _____

_____

_____

_____

20__: _____

_____

_____

_____

INTERPERSONAL – Toxic
relationships can ruin your health, while
loving relationships boost your well-
being. Choose the best, leave the rest.

FEBRUARY 24

We do not see things as they are, we see things as we are.
Anais Win

20__: _____

_____

_____

_____

20__: _____

_____

_____

_____

20__: _____

_____

_____

_____

OUTLOOK – Attitude influences outcome. Your outlook can impact the progression of disease or the increase of health. Choose to stay positive today.

FEBRUARY 25

Chocolate is not a food group—but is okay once in a while.
Walt Larimore, MD

20__: _____

_____

_____

_____

20__: _____

_____

_____

_____

20__: _____

_____

_____

_____

NUTRITION – Food is the fuel that drives your life. It can rev you up or slow you down. Evaluate your intake. Eat for energy. Eat for life!

FEBRUARY 26

. . . .

When people make personal commitments to make wiser choices,
to enjoy adequate rest, to celebrate the best in their
environment, and more—amazing things happen.
Des Cummings Jr., PhD

20__: _____

_____

_____

_____

20__: _____

_____

_____

_____

20__: _____

_____

_____

_____

CHOICE – First we make choices,
then choices make us. Choose an
inspiring destination, then create a set
of healthy habits to get you there.

FEBRUARY 27

*"TIME OUT!" Catch your breath, rethink strategy,
and jump back in the game.*
Art Bakewell

20__: _____

_____

_____

_____

20__: _____

_____

_____

_____

20__: _____

_____

_____

_____

REST – Rest rebuilds the mind, body,
and spirit. The best rest includes a
sanctuary of time set aside to rejuvenate
daily, weekly, and annually.

FEBRUARY 28

....

*We have houses, electricity, plumbing, heat ... maybe we're so
sheltered and comfortable that we've lost touch with the
natural world and forgotten our place in it.*
Bill Watterson

20__: _____

_____

_____

_____

20__: _____

_____

_____

_____

20__: _____

_____

_____

_____

E **ENVIRONMENT** – All of your
senses—sight, smell, sound, touch, and
taste—influence your mood and your
health. So optimize your environment.

FEBRUARY 29

*It does not matter how slow you go
so long as you do not stop.*
Confucius

20__: _____

_____

_____

_____

20__: _____

_____

_____

_____

20__: _____

_____

_____

_____

ACTIVITY – Activity includes both
mental and physical strengthening. A fit
mind promotes a healthy body, and a
healthy body promotes a fit mind.

MARCH 1

. . . .

God cannot give us a happiness and peace apart from himself,
because it is not there. There is no such thing.
C.S. Lewis

20__: _____

_____

_____

_____

20__: _____

_____

_____

_____

20__: _____

_____

_____

_____

TRUST – Trust in God can promote
better health. Faith, hope, and love
provide lasting peace and may help you
live a longer, happier life.

MARCH 2

A little consideration, a little thought for
others makes all the difference.
A.A. Milne

20__: _____

_____

_____

_____

20__: _____

_____

_____

_____

20__: _____

_____

_____

_____

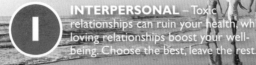

INTERPERSONAL – Toxic
relationships can ruin your health, while
loving relationships boost your well-
being. Choose the best, leave the rest.

MARCH 3

. . . .

Nothing is impossible, the word itself says, "I'm possible."
Audrey Hepburn

20__: _____

_____

_____

_____

20__: _____

_____

_____

_____

20__: _____

_____

_____

_____

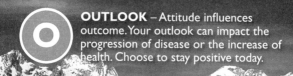

OUTLOOK – Attitude influences outcome. Your outlook can impact the progression of disease or the increase of health. Choose to stay positive today.

MARCH 4

. . . .

If you can't pronounce it, don't eat it.
Unknown

20___: _____

_____

_____

_____

20___: _____

_____

_____

_____

20___: _____

_____

_____

_____

NUTRITION – Food is the fuel that drives your life. It can rev you up or slow you down. Evaluate your intake. Eat for energy. Eat for life!

MARCH 5

. . . .

*In any moment of decision, the best thing you
can do is the right thing. The worst
thing you can do is nothing.*
Theodore Roosevelt

20__: _____

_____

_____

_____

20__: _____

_____

_____

_____

20__: _____

_____

_____

_____

CHOICE – First we make choices,
then choices make us. Choose an
inspiring destination, then create a set
of healthy habits to get you there.

MARCH 6

. . . .

I count it as a certainty that in paradise, everyone naps.
Tom Hodgkinson

20__: _____

_____

_____

_____

20__: _____

_____

_____

_____

20__: _____

_____

_____

_____

REST – Rest rebuilds the mind, body, and spirit. The best rest includes a sanctuary of time set aside to rejuvenate daily, weekly, and annually.

MARCH 7

. . . .

*Environment is the natural setting where
you find peace and healing.*
Monica Reed, MD

20__: _____

_____

_____

_____

20__: _____

_____

_____

_____

20__: _____

_____

_____

_____

E **ENVIRONMENT** – All of your
senses—sight, smell, sound, touch, and
taste—influence your mood and your
health. So optimize your environment.

MARCH 8

. . . .

For exercise, I now run with my chocolate Lab puppy, Oscar.
Daniela Pestova

20__: _____

_____

_____

_____

20__: _____

_____

_____

_____

20__: _____

_____

_____

_____

ACTIVITY – Activity includes both mental and physical strengthening. A fit mind promotes a healthy body, and a healthy body promotes a fit mind.

MARCH 9

*After spending time alone with God, we find that he injects
into our bodies energy, power, and strength.*
Charles Stanley

20__: _____

_____

_____

_____

20__: _____

_____

_____

_____

20__: _____

_____

_____

_____

TRUST – Trust in God can promote
better health. Faith, hope, and love
provide lasting peace and may help you
live a longer, happier life.

MARCH 10

. . . .

*I have loved, and I have been loved. All the
rest is just background music.*
Estelle Ramey

20__: _____
_____
_____
_____

20__: _____
_____
_____
_____

20__: _____
_____
_____
_____

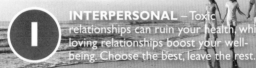

INTERPERSONAL – Toxic
relationships can ruin your health, while
loving relationships boost your well-
being. Choose the best, leave the rest.

MARCH 11

. . . .

For beautiful eyes, look for the good in others. For beautiful lips,
speak only words of kindness. And for poise, walk with
the knowledge that you are never alone.
Audrey Hepburn

20__: _____

_____

_____

_____

20__: _____

_____

_____

_____

20__: _____

_____

_____

_____

OUTLOOK – Attitude influences
outcome. Your outlook can impact the
progression of disease or the increase of
health. Choose to stay positive today.

MARCH 12

*Nobody can be in good health if he does not have
all the time, fresh air, sunshine, and good water.*
Chief Flying Hawk, Oglala Sioux

20__: _____

_____

_____

_____

20__: _____

_____

_____

_____

20__: _____

_____

_____

_____

NUTRITION – Food is the fuel that
drives your life. It can rev you up or slow
you down. Evaluate your intake. Eat for
energy. Eat for life!

MARCH 13

. . . .

*Difficult circumstances bring us to moment-by-moment
decisions—critical junctions in life's journey.*
Linda Nordyke Hambleton

20__: _____

_____

_____

_____

20__: _____

_____

_____

_____

20__: _____

_____

_____

_____

CHOICE – First we make choices,
then choices make us. Choose an
inspiring destination, then create a set
of healthy habits to get you there.

MARCH 14

. . . .

*Rest can come as a 10-minute power nap, a 20-second
mini-vacation, or eight hours of wonderful sleep.*
Des Cummings Jr., PhD

20__: _____

_____

_____

_____

20__: _____

_____

_____

_____

20__: _____

_____

_____

_____

REST – Rest rebuilds the mind, body,
and spirit. The best rest includes a
sanctuary of time set aside to rejuvenate
daily, weekly, and annually.

MARCH 15

. . . .

*And this, our life, exempt from public haunt, finds tongues
in trees, books in the running brooks, sermons
in stones, and good in everything.*
William Shakespeare

20__: _____

_____

_____

_____

20__: _____

_____

_____

_____

20__: _____

_____

_____

_____

E **ENVIRONMENT** – All of your
senses—sight, smell, sound, touch, and
taste—influence your mood and your
health. So optimize your environment.

MARCH 16

*Physical fitness is not only one of the most important keys
to a healthy body, it is the basis of dynamic
and creative intellectual activity.*
John F. Kennedy

20__: _____

_____

_____

_____

20__: _____

_____

_____

_____

20__: _____

_____

_____

_____

ACTIVITY – Activity includes both
mental and physical strengthening. A fit
mind promotes a healthy body, and a
healthy body promotes a fit mind.

MARCH 17

Never be afraid to trust an unknown future to a known God.
Corrie Ten Boom

20__: _____

_____

_____

20__: _____

_____

_____

20__: _____

_____

_____

_____

TRUST – Trust in God can promote better health. Faith, hope, and love provide lasting peace and may help you live a longer, happier life.

MARCH 18

*Friendship, like the immortality of the
soul, is too good to be believed.*
Ralph Waldo Emerson

20__: _____

_____

_____

_____

20__: _____

_____

_____

_____

20__: _____

_____

_____

_____

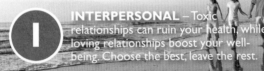

I

INTERPERSONAL – Toxic
relationships can ruin your health, while
loving relationships boost your well-
being. Choose the best, leave the rest.

MARCH 19

. . . .

Between now and bedtime ... each moment I
should be able to say, "I'm having the
time of my life right now."
Bill Watterson

20___: _____

_____

_____

_____

20___: _____

_____

_____

_____

20___: _____

_____

_____

_____

OUTLOOK – Attitude influences
outcome. Your outlook can impact the
progression of disease or the increase of
health. Choose to stay positive today.

MARCH 20

. . . .

God has provided us with a varied and rich abundance of incredibly
tasty fruits, grains, nuts, and vegetables, all of which meet or
exceed our dietary needs and keep us fit and healthy.
Clifford Goldstein

20___: _____

_____

_____

_____

20___: _____

_____

_____

_____

20___: _____

_____

_____

_____

NUTRITION – Food is the fuel that
drives your life. It can rev you up or slow
you down. Evaluate your intake. Eat for
energy. Eat for life!

MARCH 21

Who are those who fear the LORD? He will show them the path they should choose.
Psalm 25:12

20__: _____

_____

_____

_____

20__: _____

_____

_____

_____

20__: _____

_____

_____

_____

CHOICE – First we make choices, then choices make us. Choose an inspiring destination, then create a set of healthy habits to get you there.

MARCH 22

*Rest replaces weariness, exhaustion, and
fatigue with peace, energy, and hope.*
Des Cummings Jr., PhD

20__: _____

_____

_____

_____

20__: _____

_____

_____

_____

20__: _____

_____

_____

_____

REST – Rest rebuilds the mind, body,
and spirit. The best rest includes a
sanctuary of time set aside to rejuvenate
daily, weekly, and annually.

MARCH 23

. . . .

Get out there.
Brunton Company

20__: _____

_____

_____

_____

20__: _____

_____

_____

_____

20__: _____

_____

_____

_____

ENVIRONMENT – All of your
senses—sight, smell, sound, touch, and
taste—influence your mood and your
health. So optimize your environment.

MARCH 24

....

*The Lord God took the man and put him in
the Garden of Eden to work it
and take care of it.*
Genesis 2:15

20__: _____

_____

_____

_____

20__: _____

_____

_____

_____

20__: _____

_____

_____

_____

ACTIVITY – Activity includes both
mental and physical strengthening. A fit
mind promotes a healthy body, and a
healthy body promotes a fit mind.

MARCH 25

. . . .

*Every experience God gives us, every person he puts
into our lives, is the perfect preparation for
a future only he can see.*
Corrie Ten Boom

20__: _____

_____

_____

_____

20__: _____

_____

_____

_____

20__: _____

_____

_____

_____

TRUST – Trust in God can promote
better health. Faith, hope, and love
provide lasting peace and may help you
live a longer, happier life.

MARCH 26

I love you, not for what you are, but for
what I am when I am with you.
Roy Croft

20__: _____

_____

_____

_____

20__: _____

_____

_____

_____

20__: _____

_____

_____

_____

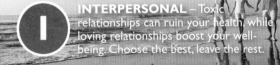

I

INTERPERSONAL – Toxic
relationships can ruin your health, while
loving relationships boost your well-
being. Choose the best, leave the rest.

MARCH 27

. . . .

*To make a bad day worse, spend it
wishing for the impossible.*
Bill Watterson

20__: _____

_____

_____

_____

20__: _____

_____

_____

_____

20__: _____

_____

_____

_____

OUTLOOK – Attitude influences
outcome. Your outlook can impact the
progression of disease or the increase of
health. Choose to stay positive today.

MARCH 28

. . . .

A healthful lifestyle, one based on the simple principles of natural law and sound medical science, can go a long way in not only making our lives here better, but longer, as well.

Clifford Goldstein

20__: _____

_____

_____

_____

20__: _____

_____

_____

_____

20__: _____

_____

_____

_____

NUTRITION – Food is the fuel that drives your life. It can rev you up or slow you down. Evaluate your intake. Eat for energy. Eat for life!

MARCH 29

Choose my instruction instead of silver,
knowledge rather than choice gold.
Proverbs 8:10

20__: _____

_____

_____

_____

20__: _____

_____

_____

_____

20__: _____

_____

_____

_____

CHOICE – First we make choices,
then choices make us. Choose an
inspiring destination, then create a set
of healthy habits to get you there.

MARCH 30

God's healing rest is as close as the beating of your heart.
Des Cummings Jr., PhD

20__: _____

_____

_____

_____

20__: _____

_____

_____

_____

20__: _____

_____

_____

_____

REST – Rest rebuilds the mind, body, and spirit. The best rest includes a sanctuary of time set aside to rejuvenate daily, weekly, and annually.

MARCH 31

. . . .

*We know that God is everywhere; but certainly we feel
his presence most when his works are on the
grandest scale spread before us ...*
Charlotte Bronte

20__: _____

_____

_____

_____

20__: _____

_____

_____

_____

20__: _____

_____

_____

_____

E **ENVIRONMENT** – All of your
senses—sight, smell, sound, touch, and
taste—influence your mood and your
health. So optimize your environment.

APRIL 1

....

*Our growing softness, our increasing lack of physical
fitness, is a menace to our security.*
John F. Kennedy

20__: _____

_____

_____

_____

20__: _____

_____

_____

_____

20__: _____

_____

_____

_____

ACTIVITY – Activity includes both
mental and physical strengthening. A fit
mind promotes a healthy body, and a
healthy body promotes a fit mind.

APRIL 2

Trust in the Lord with all your heart, and lean not on your own understanding; In all your ways, acknowledge Him, and He shall direct your paths.
Proverbs 3:5-6 (NKJV)

20__: _____

_____

_____

_____

20__: _____

_____

_____

_____

20__: _____

_____

_____

_____

TRUST – Trust in God can promote better health. Faith, hope, and love provide lasting peace and may help you live a longer, happier life.

APRIL 3

. . . .

Friendships win at home, at work, and play for all
of life and throughout all of eternity.
Des Cummings Jr., PhD

20__: _____

_____

_____

_____

20__: _____

_____

_____

_____

20__: _____

_____

_____

_____

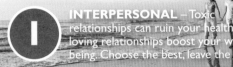

INTERPERSONAL – Toxic
relationships can ruin your health, while
loving relationships boost your well-
being. Choose the best, leave the rest.

APRIL 4

. . . .

*We're so busy watching out for what's just
ahead of us that we don't take time
to enjoy where we are.*
Bill Watterson

20__: _____

_____

_____

_____

20__: _____

_____

_____

_____

20__: _____

_____

_____

_____

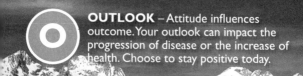

OUTLOOK – Attitude influences
outcome. Your outlook can impact the
progression of disease or the increase of
health. Choose to stay positive today.

APRIL 5

....

*Test us for ten days, [Daniel] said. Give us
vegetables to eat and water to drink.*
Daniel 1:12 (GNT)

20__: _____

_____

_____

20__: _____

_____

_____

_____

20__: _____

_____

_____

_____

NUTRITION – Food is the fuel that
drives your life. It can rev you up or slow
you down. Evaluate your intake. Eat for
energy. Eat for life!

APRIL 6

It all boils down to a choice, doesn't it?
Dr. Dick Tibbits

20__: _____

_____

_____

_____

20__: _____

_____

_____

_____

20__: _____

_____

_____

_____

CHOICE – First we make choices, then choices make us. Choose an inspiring destination, then create a set of healthy habits to get you there.

APRIL 7

We are such stuff as dreams are made on, and
our little life is rounded with a sleep.
William Shakespeare

20___: _____

_____

_____

_____

20___: _____

_____

_____

_____

20___: _____

_____

_____

_____

REST – Rest rebuilds the mind, body, and spirit. The best rest includes a sanctuary of time set aside to rejuvenate daily, weekly, and annually.

APRIL 8

The world is mud-luscious and puddle-wonderful.
e.e. cummings

20__: _____

_____

_____

20__: _____

_____

_____

20__: _____

_____

_____

ENVIRONMENT – All of your senses—sight, smell, sound, touch, and taste—influence your mood and your health. So optimize your environment.

APRIL 9

....

*Methinks that the moment my legs begin to
move, my thoughts begin to flow.*
Henry David Thoreau

20__: _____

_____

_____

_____

20__: _____

_____

_____

_____

20__: _____

_____

_____

_____

ACTIVITY – Activity includes both
mental and physical strengthening. A fit
mind promotes a healthy body, and a
healthy body promotes a fit mind.

APRIL 10

....

I believe in Christ like I believe in the sun—
not because I can see it, but by it
I can see everything else.
C.S. Lewis

20__: _____

_____

_____

_____

20__: _____

_____

_____

_____

20__: _____

_____

_____

_____

TRUST – Trust in God can promote
better health. Faith, hope, and love
provide lasting peace and may help you
live a longer, happier life.

APRIL 11

. . . .

God gave you a gift of 86,400 seconds today.
Have you used one to say "thank you?"
William A. Ward

20__: _____

_____

_____

_____

20__: _____

_____

_____

_____

20__: _____

_____

_____

_____

I **INTERPERSONAL** – Toxic relationships can ruin your health, while loving relationships boost your well-being. Choose the best, leave the rest.

APRIL 12

....

The opposite of play is not ... work ... it is depression.
Brian Sutton-Smith

20__: _____

_____

_____

_____

20__: _____

_____

_____

_____

20__: _____

_____

_____

_____

OUTLOOK – Attitude influences
outcome. Your outlook can impact the
progression of disease or the increase of
health. Choose to stay positive today.

APRIL 13

....

Food ... is the first wealth. Grow it right, and you feel insanely rich, no matter what you own.
Kristin Kimball

20__: _____

_____

_____

_____

20__: _____

_____

_____

_____

20__: _____

_____

_____

_____

NUTRITION – Food is the fuel that drives your life. It can rev you up or slow you down. Evaluate your intake. Eat for energy. Eat for life!

APRIL 14

. . . .

And who wouldn't choose to live with a bright optimism
about the future rather than a dark
pessimism about the past?
Dr. Dick Tibbits

20__: _____

_____

_____

_____

20__: _____

_____

_____

_____

20__: _____

_____

_____

_____

CHOICE – First we make choices,
then choices make us. Choose an
inspiring destination, then create a set
of healthy habits to get you there.

APRIL 15

True silence is the rest of the mind, and is to the spirit what sleep is to the body, nourishment and refreshment.
William Penn

20__: _____

_____

_____

_____

20__: _____

_____

_____

_____

20__: _____

_____

_____

_____

REST – Rest rebuilds the mind, body, and spirit. The best rest includes a sanctuary of time set aside to rejuvenate daily, weekly, and annually.

APRIL 16

. . . .

Be careful the environment you choose for it will shape you.
W. Clement Stone

20__: _____

_____

_____

_____

20__: _____

_____

_____

_____

20__: _____

_____

_____

_____

E **ENVIRONMENT** – All of your senses—sight, smell, sound, touch, and taste—influence your mood and your health. So optimize your environment.

APRIL 17

Activity is how we experience the power of life.
Des Cummings Jr., PhD

20__: _____

_____

_____

_____

20__: _____

_____

_____

_____

20__: _____

_____

_____

_____

ACTIVITY – Activity includes both mental and physical strengthening. A fit mind promotes a healthy body, and a healthy body promotes a fit mind.

APRIL 18

. . . .

*As we reflect, we draw upon our values, morals, and
core beliefs about what is right and true.*
Dr. Dick Tibbits

20__: _____

_____

_____

_____

20__: _____

_____

_____

_____

20__: _____

_____

_____

_____

TRUST – Trust in God can promote
better health. Faith, hope, and love
provide lasting peace and may help you
live a longer, happier life.

APRIL 19

Every day I need the forgiveness of the persons I may hurt by even my best decisions. Every day I need the forgiveness of those who care for these persons. And every day I need to forgive myself.
Sandy Shugart, PhD

20__: _____

_____

_____

_____

20__: _____

_____

_____

_____

20__: _____

_____

_____

_____

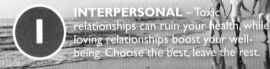

INTERPERSONAL – Toxic relationships can ruin your health, while loving relationships boost your well-being. Choose the best, leave the rest.

APRIL 20

. . . .

Set your minds on things above, not on earthly
things. For you died, and your life is
now hidden with Christ in God.
Colossians 3:2-3 (NIV)

20__: _____

_____

_____

_____

20__: _____

_____

_____

_____

20__: _____

_____

_____

_____

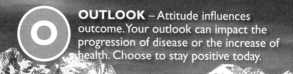

OUTLOOK – Attitude influences
outcome. Your outlook can impact the
progression of disease or the increase of
health. Choose to stay positive today.

APRIL 21

A man too busy to take care of his health is like a
mechanic too busy to take care of his tools.
Spanish Proverb

20___: _____

_____

_____

_____

20___: _____

_____

_____

_____

20___: _____

_____

_____

_____

NUTRITION – Food is the fuel that
drives your life. It can rev you up or slow
you down. Evaluate your intake. Eat for
energy. Eat for life!

APRIL 22

. . . .

Human beings, by changing the inner attitudes of their minds,
can change the outer aspects of their lives.
William James

20__: _____

_____

_____

_____

20__: _____

_____

_____

_____

20__: _____

_____

_____

_____

CHOICE – First we make choices,
then choices make us. Choose an
inspiring destination, then create a set
of healthy habits to get you there.

APRIL 23

. . . .

Early to bed, early to rise, makes a man
healthy, wealthy, and wise.
Benjamin Franklin

20__: _____

_____

_____

_____

20__: _____

_____

_____

_____

20__: _____

_____

_____

_____

REST – Rest rebuilds the mind, body, and spirit. The best rest includes a sanctuary of time set aside to rejuvenate daily, weekly, and annually.

APRIL 24

*I love to think of nature as an unlimited broadcasting
station, through which God speaks to us
every hour, if we will only tune in.*
George Washington Carver

20___: _____

_____

_____

_____

20___: _____

_____

_____

_____

20___: _____

_____

_____

_____

E **ENVIRONMENT** – All of your
senses—sight, smell, sound, touch, and
taste—influence your mood and your
health. So optimize your environment.

APRIL 25

....

An early morning walk is a blessing for the whole day.
Henry David Thoreau

20__: _____

_____

_____

_____

20__: _____

_____

_____

_____

20__: _____

_____

_____

_____

A **ACTIVITY** – Activity includes both mental and physical strengthening. A fit mind promotes a healthy body, and a healthy body promotes a fit mind.

APRIL 26

....

*I know that he is, but figuring out
what he is doing is another story.*
Linda Nordyke Hambleton

20__: _____

_____

_____

_____

20__: _____

_____

_____

_____

20__: _____

_____

_____

_____

TRUST – Trust in God can promote
better health. Faith, hope, and love
provide lasting peace and may help you
live a longer, happier life.

APRIL 27

Be curious, not judgmental.
Walt Whitman

20__: _____

_____

_____

_____

20__: _____

_____

_____

_____

20__: _____

_____

_____

_____

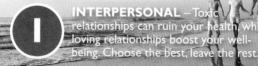

I

INTERPERSONAL – Toxic relationships can ruin your health, while loving relationships boost your well-being. Choose the best, leave the rest.

APRIL 28

....

Joy and temperance and repose
Slam the door on the doctor's nose.
Henry Wadsworth Longfellow

20__: _____

_____

_____

_____

20__: _____

_____

_____

_____

20__: _____

_____

_____

_____

OUTLOOK – Attitude influences outcome. Your outlook can impact the progression of disease or the increase of health. Choose to stay positive today.

APRIL 29

. . . .

Let food be thy medicine, and medicine thy food.
Hippocrates

20__: _____

_____

_____

_____

20__: _____

_____

_____

_____

20__: _____

_____

_____

_____

NUTRITION – Food is the fuel that drives your life. It can rev you up or slow you down. Evaluate your intake. Eat for energy. Eat for life!

APRIL 30

. . . .

Choosing with thought and intention is your greatest power.
Monica Reed, MD

20__: _____

_____

_____

_____

20__: _____

_____

_____

_____

20__: _____

_____

_____

_____

CHOICE – First we make choices, then choices make us. Choose an inspiring destination, then create a set of healthy habits to get you there.

MAY 1

*Often Jesus would walk off into the hills, or away down the beach,
where he would sit for hours . . . thinking . . . praying . . .
resting . . . sitting. . . . Preparing.*
Dick Duerksen

20__: _____

_____

_____

_____

20__: _____

_____

_____

_____

20__: _____

_____

_____

_____

REST – Rest rebuilds the mind, body,
and spirit. The best rest includes a
sanctuary of time set aside to rejuvenate
daily, weekly, and annually.

MAY 2

. . . .

Scents associated with natural things—flowers, fresh air, the sea—
tend to have a soothing effect on most people because those
aromas take them ... to a garden, a mountain retreat,
or a beautiful beach. Dr. Dick Tibbits

20__: _____

_____

_____

_____

20__: _____

_____

_____

_____

20__: _____

_____

_____

_____

E **ENVIRONMENT** – All of your
senses—sight, smell, sound, touch, and
taste—influence your mood and your
health. So optimize your environment.

MAY 3

. . . .

*People who engage in regular aerobic exercise
report better mental health and a reduced
response to stressful life events.*
Christopher Peterson

20__: _____

_____

_____

_____

20__: _____

_____

_____

_____

20__: _____

_____

_____

_____

ACTIVITY –Activity includes both
mental and physical strengthening. A fit
mind promotes a healthy body, and a
healthy body promotes a fit mind.

MAY 4

....

Fight all your battles on your knees and you win every time.
Dr. Charles Stanley

20__: _____

_____

_____

_____

20__: _____

_____

_____

_____

20__: _____

_____

_____

_____

TRUST – Trust in God can promote better health. Faith, hope, and love provide lasting peace and may help you live a longer, happier life.

MAY 5

. . . .

Your family is most blessed by the affirmation of your love.
Des Cummings Jr., PhD

20__: _____

_____

_____

_____

20__: _____

_____

_____

_____

20__: _____

_____

_____

_____

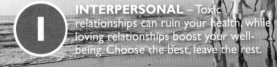

INTERPERSONAL – Toxic relationships can ruin your health, while loving relationships boost your well-being. Choose the best, leave the rest.

MAY 6

....

*If you think you can, you can; if you think you can't,
you can't. Either way, you're right.*
Henry Ford

20__: _____

_____

_____

_____

20__: _____

_____

_____

_____

20__: _____

_____

_____

_____

OUTLOOK – Attitude influences
outcome. Your outlook can impact the
progression of disease or the increase of
health. Choose to stay positive today.

MAY 7

. . . .

*The doctor of the future will no longer treat the human
frame with drugs, but rather will cure and
prevent disease with nutrition.*
Thomas Edison

20__: _____

_____

_____

_____

20__: _____

_____

_____

_____

20__: _____

_____

_____

_____

NUTRITION – Food is the fuel that
drives your life. It can rev you up or slow
you down. Evaluate your intake. Eat for
energy. Eat for life!

MAY 8

. . . .

Every accomplishment starts with the decision to try.
Gail Devers

20__: _____

_____

_____

_____

20__: _____

_____

_____

_____

20__: _____

_____

_____

_____

CHOICE – First we make choices, then choices make us. Choose an inspiring destination, then create a set of healthy habits to get you there.

MAY 9

Don't underestimate the value of doing nothing,
of just going along, listening to all the things
you can't hear, and not bothering.
A.A. Milne

20__: _____

_____

_____

_____

20__: _____

_____

_____

_____

20__: _____

_____

_____

_____

REST – Rest rebuilds the mind, body,
and spirit. The best rest includes a
sanctuary of time set aside to rejuvenate
daily, weekly, and annually.

MAY 10

. . . .

*Imagine walking through the Garden of Eden before
Adam and Eve ate of the forbidden fruit.*
Dr. Dick Tibbits

20__: _____

_____

_____

_____

20__: _____

_____

_____

_____

20__: _____

_____

_____

_____

E **ENVIRONMENT** – All of your
senses—sight, smell, sound, touch, and
taste—influence your mood and your
health. So optimize your environment.

MAY 11

. . . .

*True enjoyment comes from activity of the mind and
exercise of the body; the two are ever united.*
Wilhelm Von Humboldt

20__: _____

_____

_____

_____

20__: _____

_____

_____

_____

20__: _____

_____

_____

_____

ACTIVITY – Activity includes both
mental and physical strengthening. A fit
mind promotes a healthy body, and a
healthy body promotes a fit mind.

MAY 12

. . . .

Keep trusting God; he is always in control even when your
circumstances may seem out of control!
Unknown

20__: _____

_____

_____

_____

20__: _____

_____

_____

_____

20__: _____

_____

_____

_____

TRUST – Trust in God can promote
better health. Faith, hope, and love
provide lasting peace and may help you
live a longer, happier life.

MAY 13

. . . .

*The #1 evangelistic tool in America today is a successful
marriage, because it's a living miracle.*
Dr. Joe Aldrich

20__: _____

_____

_____

_____

20__: _____

_____

_____

_____

20__: _____

_____

_____

_____

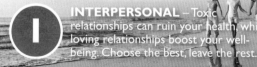

I **INTERPERSONAL** – Toxic
relationships can ruin your health, while
loving relationships boost your well-
being. Choose the best, leave the rest.

MAY 14

. . . .

Positive emotions have their greatest effect
when we stop to celebrate them!
Des Cummings Jr., PhD

20__: _____

_____

_____

_____

20__: _____

_____

_____

_____

20__: _____

_____

_____

_____

OUTLOOK – Attitude influences
outcome. Your outlook can impact the
progression of disease or the increase of
health. Choose to stay positive today.

MAY 15

....

*Then God said, "I give you every seed-bearing plant on the
face of the whole earth and every tree that has fruit
with seed in it. They will be yours for food."*
Genesis 1:29 (NIV)

20__: _____

_____

_____

_____

20__: _____

_____

_____

_____

20__: _____

_____

_____

_____

NUTRITION – Food is the fuel that
drives your life. It can rev you up or slow
you down. Evaluate your intake. Eat for
energy. Eat for life!

MAY 16

. . . .

People inspire you or they drain you—pick them wisely.
Hans F. Hansen

20__: _____

_____

_____

_____

20__: _____

_____

_____

_____

20__: _____

_____

_____

_____

CHOICE – First we make choices, then choices make us. Choose an inspiring destination, then create a set of healthy habits to get you there.

MAY 17

. . . .

*It is important to note that we were not made for
this. Our bodies are not adapted to an
environment of sustained stress.*
Sandy Shugart, PhD

20__: _____

_____

_____

_____

20__: _____

_____

_____

_____

20__: _____

_____

_____

_____

REST – Rest rebuilds the mind, body,
and spirit. The best rest includes a
sanctuary of time set aside to rejuvenate
daily, weekly, and annually.

MAY 18

Earth laughs in flowers.
Ralph Waldo Emerson

20__: _____

_____

_____

_____

20__: _____

_____

_____

_____

20__: _____

_____

_____

_____

ENVIRONMENT – All of your senses—sight, smell, sound, touch, and taste—influence your mood and your health. So optimize your environment.

MAY 19

Staying physically fit is the fountain of youth.
Monica Reed, MD

20__: _____

_____

_____

_____

20__: _____

_____

_____

_____

20__: _____

_____

_____

_____

ACTIVITY – Activity includes both mental and physical strengthening. A fit mind promotes a healthy body, and a healthy body promotes a fit mind.

MAY 20

. . . .

Worry implies that we don't quite trust that God is big enough,
powerful enough, or loving enough to take care of
what's happening in our lives.
Francis Chan

20__: _____

_____

_____

_____

20__: _____

_____

_____

_____

20__: _____

_____

_____

_____

TRUST – Trust in God can promote
better health. Faith, hope, and love
provide lasting peace and may help you
live a longer, happier life.

MAY 21

. . . .

The family meal may be a lost art,
but it's well worth recovering.
Walt Larimore, MD

20__: _____

_____

_____

_____

20__: _____

_____

_____

_____

20__: _____

_____

_____

_____

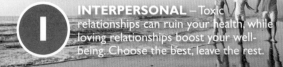

INTERPERSONAL – Toxic
relationships can ruin your health, while
loving relationships boost your well-
being. Choose the best, leave the rest.

MAY 22

. . . .

A cheerful heart does good like medicine,
but a broken spirit makes one sick.
Proverbs 17:22 (TLB)

20__: _____

_____

_____

_____

20__: _____

_____

_____

_____

20__: _____

_____

_____

_____

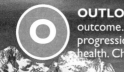

OUTLOOK – Attitude influences
outcome. Your outlook can impact the
progression of disease or the increase of
health. Choose to stay positive today.

MAY 23

Their fruit will be for food and their leaves for medicine.
Ezekiel 47:12 (NKJV)

20__: _____

_____

_____

_____

20__: _____

_____

_____

_____

20__: _____

_____

_____

_____

NUTRITION – Food is the fuel that drives your life. It can rev you up or slow you down. Evaluate your intake. Eat for energy. Eat for life!

MAY 24

. . . .

*Every tomorrow has two handles. We can take hold of it
with the handle of anxiety or the handle of faith.*
Henry Ward Beecher

20__: _____

_____

_____

_____

20__: _____

_____

_____

_____

20__: _____

_____

_____

_____

CHOICE – First we make choices,
then choices make us. Choose an
inspiring destination, then create a set
of healthy habits to get you there.

MAY 25

Our lives were meant for calm, not chaos.
Thomas Kinkade

20__: _____

_____

_____

_____

20__: _____

_____

_____

_____

20__: _____

_____

_____

_____

REST – Rest rebuilds the mind, body, and spirit. The best rest includes a sanctuary of time set aside to rejuvenate daily, weekly, and annually.

MAY 26

. . . .

Along with milk and vegetables, kids need
a steady diet of rocks and worms.
Unknown

20__: _____

_____

_____

_____

20__: _____

_____

_____

_____

20__: _____

_____

_____

_____

E **ENVIRONMENT** – All of your
senses—sight, smell, sound, touch, and
taste—influence your mood and your
health. So optimize your environment.

MAY 27

*Physical activity is an excellent stress-buster and provides
other health benefits as well. It can also improve
your mood and self-image.*
Jon Wickham

20__: _____

_____

_____

_____

20__: _____

_____

_____

_____

20__: _____

_____

_____

_____

ACTIVITY – Activity includes both
mental and physical strengthening. A fit
mind promotes a healthy body, and a
healthy body promotes a fit mind.

MAY 28

. . . .

Joseph woke up in a prison but went to sleep in a palace the very same night. Why? Because he trusted God in his dungeon. Trust God no matter where you find yourself today. He will take care of you. Anna Bachinsky

20__: _____

_____

_____

_____

20__: _____

_____

_____

_____

20__: _____

_____

_____

_____

TRUST – Trust in God can promote better health. Faith, hope, and love provide lasting peace and may help you live a longer, happier life.

MAY 29

. . . .

*If it wasn't good for Adam to be alone,
why would it be good for us now?*
Monica Reed, MD

20__: _____

_____

_____

_____

20__: _____

_____

_____

_____

20__: _____

_____

_____

_____

INTERPERSONAL – Toxic
relationships can ruin your health, while
loving relationships boost your well-
being. Choose the best, leave the rest.

MAY 30

. . . .

If people sat outside and looked at the stars each night,
I'll bet they'd live a lot differently.
Bill Watterson

20__: _____

_____

_____

_____

20__: _____

_____

_____

_____

20__: _____

_____

_____

_____

OUTLOOK – Attitude influences outcome. Your outlook can impact the progression of disease or the increase of health. Choose to stay positive today.

MAY 31

....

A man may esteem himself happy when that
which is his food is also his medicine.
Henry David Thoreau

20__: _____

_____

_____

_____

20__: _____

_____

_____

_____

20__: _____

_____

_____

_____

NUTRITION – Food is the fuel that
drives your life. It can rev you up or slow
you down. Evaluate your intake. Eat for
energy. Eat for life!

JUNE 1

. . . .

No matter what your health history, you can choose today to
make better, more consistent choices tomorrow.
Des Cummings Jr., PhD

20__: _____

_____

_____

_____

20__: _____

_____

_____

_____

20__: _____

_____

_____

_____

CHOICE – First we make choices,
then choices make us. Choose an
inspiring destination, then create a set
of healthy habits to get you there.

JUNE 2

Sabbath makes the other days of my week doable.
Monica Reed, MD

20__: _____

_____

_____

_____

20__: _____

_____

_____

_____

20__: _____

_____

_____

_____

REST – Rest rebuilds the mind, body, and spirit. The best rest includes a sanctuary of time set aside to rejuvenate daily, weekly, and annually.

JUNE 3

. . . .

*Everybody needs beauty as well as bread, places to play
in and pray in, where nature may heal and
give strength to body and soul.*
John Muir

20__: _____

_____

_____

_____

20__: _____

_____

_____

_____

20__: _____

_____

_____

_____

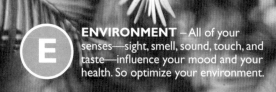

E **ENVIRONMENT** – All of your
senses—sight, smell, sound, touch, and
taste—influence your mood and your
health. So optimize your environment.

JUNE 4

. . . .

Investing in health will produce enormous benefits.
G.H. Brundtland

20__: _____

_____

_____

_____

20__: _____

_____

_____

_____

20__: _____

_____

_____

_____

ACTIVITY – Activity includes both
mental and physical strengthening. A fit
mind promotes a healthy body, and a
healthy body promotes a fit mind.

JUNE 5

. . . .

I have learned that faith means trusting in advance
what will only make sense in reverse.
Philip Yancey

20__: _____

_____

_____

_____

20__: _____

_____

_____

_____

20__: _____

_____

_____

_____

_____

TRUST – Trust in God can promote
better health. Faith, hope, and love
provide lasting peace and may help you
live a longer, happier life.

JUNE 6

. . . .

*Let us think of ways to motivate one another
to acts of love and good works.*
Hebrews 10:24

20__: _____

_____

_____

_____

20__: _____

_____

_____

_____

20__: _____

_____

_____

_____

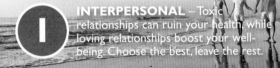

I

INTERPERSONAL – Toxic relationships can ruin your health, while loving relationships boost your well-being. Choose the best, leave the rest.

JUNE 7

. . . .

Hope is the conviction that what is happening means
something, the struggle matters, the sacrifice
and the sweat and the risk have value.
Sandy Shugart, PhD

20__: _____

_____

_____

_____

20__: _____

_____

_____

_____

20__: _____

_____

_____

_____

OUTLOOK – Attitude influences
outcome. Your outlook can impact the
progression of disease or the increase of
health. Choose to stay positive today.

JUNE 8

. . . .

*You don't have to cook fancy or complicated
masterpieces— just good food
from fresh ingredients.*
Julia Child

20__: _____

_____

_____

_____

20__: _____

_____

_____

_____

20__: _____

_____

_____

_____

NUTRITION – Food is the fuel that
drives your life. It can rev you up or slow
you down. Evaluate your intake. Eat for
energy. Eat for life!

JUNE 9

. . . .

Happiness can be found even in the darkest of times
if one only remembers to turn on the light.
J.K. Rowling

20__: _____

_____

_____

_____

20__: _____

_____

_____

_____

20__: _____

_____

_____

_____

CHOICE – First we make choices,
then choices make us. Choose an
inspiring destination, then create a set
of healthy habits to get you there.

JUNE 10

Remember the Sabbath day by keeping it holy.
On it you shall not do any work.
Exodus 20:8-10 (NIV)

20__: _____

_____

_____

_____

20__: _____

_____

_____

_____

20__: _____

_____

_____

_____

REST – Rest rebuilds the mind, body, and spirit. The best rest includes a sanctuary of time set aside to rejuvenate daily, weekly, and annually.

JUNE 11

. . . .

Short term, it would make me happy to go play outside. Long term, it would make me happier to do well at school and become successful. But in the VERY long term, I know which will make better memories. Bill Watterson

20__: _____

_____

_____

_____

20__: _____

_____

_____

_____

20__: _____

_____

_____

_____

E **ENVIRONMENT** – All of your senses—sight, smell, sound, touch, and taste—influence your mood and your health. So optimize your environment.

JUNE 12

. . . .

Spiritually, those who exercise often find a deeper
connection to their Creator, who made them
for a life of health, happiness, and peace.
Des Cummings Jr., PhD

20__: _____

_____

_____

_____

20__: _____

_____

_____

_____

20__: _____

_____

_____

_____

ACTIVITY – Activity includes both
mental and physical strengthening. A fit
mind promotes a healthy body, and a
healthy body promotes a fit mind.

JUNE 13

Belief in God is the basis of all health.
John Harvey Kellogg, MD

20__: _____

_____

_____

_____

20__: _____

_____

_____

_____

20__: _____

_____

_____

_____

TRUST – Trust in God can promote better health. Faith, hope, and love provide lasting peace and may help you live a longer, happier life.

JUNE 14

. . . .

*How much better it would be if we all could reach
across the barrier of illness and disease
and touch each other as real people!*
Linda Nordyke Hambleton

20__: _____

_____

_____

_____

20__: _____

_____

_____

_____

20__: _____

_____

_____

_____

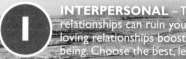

I **INTERPERSONAL** – Toxic relationships can ruin your health, while loving relationships boost your well-being. Choose the best, leave the rest.

JUNE 15

. . . .

Happiness has no time limits or conditions;
the only requirement is to give it away.
George Alexiou

20__: _____

_____

_____

_____

20__: _____

_____

_____

_____

20__: _____

_____

_____

_____

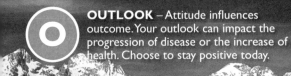

OUTLOOK – Attitude influences
outcome. Your outlook can impact the
progression of disease or the increase of
health. Choose to stay positive today.

JUNE 16

. . . .

Those who think they have no time for healthy eating
will sooner or later have to find time for illness.
Edward Stanley

20__: _____

_____

_____

_____

20__: _____

_____

_____

_____

20__: _____

_____

_____

_____

NUTRITION – Food is the fuel that drives your life. It can rev you up or slow you down. Evaluate your intake. Eat for energy. Eat for life!

JUNE 17

....

We are our choices.
Jean-Paul Sartre

20__: _____

_____

_____

_____

20__: _____

_____

_____

_____

20__: _____

_____

_____

_____

CHOICE – First we make choices,
then choices make us. Choose an
inspiring destination, then create a set
of healthy habits to get you there.

JUNE 18

...My presence will go with you and I will give you rest.
Exodus 33:14 (NIV)

20__: _____

_____

_____

_____

20__: _____

_____

_____

_____

20__: _____

_____

_____

_____

REST – Rest rebuilds the mind, body, and spirit. The best rest includes a sanctuary of time set aside to rejuvenate daily, weekly, and annually.

JUNE 19

. . . .

Color will always chase the gray away.
Unknown

20__: _____

_____

_____

_____

20__: _____

_____

_____

_____

20__: _____

_____

_____

_____

E

ENVIRONMENT – All of your
senses—sight, smell, sound, touch, and
taste—influence your mood and your
health. So optimize your environment.

JUNE 20

*Great things happen when the mind, body, and spirit
fully engage and reach a pinnacle.*
Des Cummings Jr., PhD

20__: _____

_____

_____

_____

20__: _____

_____

_____

_____

20__: _____

_____

_____

_____

ACTIVITY – Activity includes both
mental and physical strengthening. A fit
mind promotes a healthy body, and a
healthy body promotes a fit mind.

JUNE 21

. . . .

*I would rather be what God chose to make me than the most
glorious creature that I could think of; for to have been
thought about ... and then made by God, is the ...
most precious thing ...* George MacDonald

20__: _____

_____

_____

_____

20__: _____

_____

_____

_____

20__: _____

_____

_____

_____

TRUST – Trust in God can promote
better health. Faith, hope, and love
provide lasting peace and may help you
live a longer, happier life.

JUNE 22

*True friends are those who really know
you but love you anyway.*
Edna Buchannan

20__: _____

_____

_____

_____

20__: _____

_____

_____

_____

20__: _____

_____

_____

_____

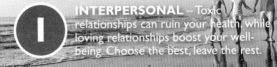

I

INTERPERSONAL – Toxic
relationships can ruin your health, while
loving relationships boost your well-
being. Choose the best, leave the rest.

JUNE 23

. . . .

*Adopting the right attitude can convert a
negative stress into a positive one.*
Dr. Hans Selye

20__: _____

_____

_____

_____

20__: _____

_____

_____

_____

20__: _____

_____

_____

_____

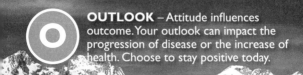

OUTLOOK – Attitude influences
outcome. Your outlook can impact the
progression of disease or the increase of
health. Choose to stay positive today.

JUNE 24

. . . .

Yes, food is serious, but you should have fun with it.
Emril Lagasse

20__: _____

_____

_____

_____

20__: _____

_____

_____

_____

20__: _____

_____

_____

_____

NUTRITION – Food is the fuel that
drives your life. It can rev you up or slow
you down. Evaluate your intake. Eat for
energy. Eat for life!

JUNE 25

*If you go, you can either win or not win. If you don't
go for it, you definitely won't win.*
Jens Voigt

20__: _____

_____

_____

_____

20__: _____

_____

_____

_____

20__: _____

_____

_____

_____

CHOICE – First we make choices,
then choices make us. Choose an
inspiring destination, then create a set
of healthy habits to get you there.

JUNE 26

....

*The less a child sleeps, the more likely
he or she is to be SuperSized!*
Sherri Flynt, MPH, RD, LD

20__: _____

_____

_____

_____

20__: _____

_____

_____

_____

20__: _____

_____

_____

_____

REST – Rest rebuilds the mind, body,
and spirit. The best rest includes a
sanctuary of time set aside to rejuvenate
daily, weekly, and annually.

JUNE 27

. . . .

When we go outside to take in the sunshine, smell the flowers,
and feel the wind on our faces or the rain on our cheeks,
we are participating in something far greater
than ourselves. Elizabeth Hulford

20___: _____

_____

_____

_____

20___: _____

_____

_____

_____

20___: _____

_____

_____

_____

E **ENVIRONMENT** – All of your
senses—sight, smell, sound, touch, and
taste—influence your mood and your
health. So optimize your environment.

JUNE 28

. . . .

Walking is a man's best friend.
Hippocrates

20__: _____

_____

_____

_____

20__: _____

_____

_____

_____

20__: _____

_____

_____

_____

ACTIVITY – Activity includes both mental and physical strengthening. A fit mind promotes a healthy body, and a healthy body promotes a fit mind.

JUNE 29

*A believer understands God can be trusted in all
circumstances—even when it isn't clear why
things happen the way they do.*
Gordon Retzer

20__: _____

_____

_____

_____

20__: _____

_____

_____

_____

20__: _____

_____

_____

_____

TRUST – Trust in God can promote
better health. Faith, hope, and love
provide lasting peace and may help you
live a longer, happier life.

JUNE 30

. . . .

If you are angry, don't sin by nursing your grudge.
Don't let the sun go down with you still
angry—get over it quickly.
Ephesians 4:26 (TLB)

20___: _____

_____

_____

_____

20___: _____

_____

_____

_____

20___: _____

_____

_____

_____

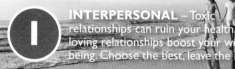

INTERPERSONAL – Toxic
relationships can ruin your health, while
loving relationships boost your well-
being. Choose the best, leave the rest.

JULY 1

....

Outlook is your ability to stay "mentally fit."
Monica Reed, MD

20__: _____

_____

_____

_____

20__: _____

_____

_____

_____

20__: _____

_____

_____

_____

OUTLOOK – Attitude influences
outcome. Your outlook can impact the
progression of disease or the increase of
health. Choose to stay positive today.

JULY 2

If you keep good food in your fridge, you will eat good food.
Errick McAdams

20__: _____

_____

_____

_____

20__: _____

_____

_____

_____

20__: _____

_____

_____

_____

NUTRITION – Food is the fuel that drives your life. It can rev you up or slow you down. Evaluate your intake. Eat for energy. Eat for life!

JULY 3

....

No, I do not accept defeat here. I do not accept this.
I'm going to change this.
Jens Voigt

20___: _____

_____

_____

_____

20___: _____

_____

_____

_____

20___: _____

_____

_____

_____

CHOICE – First we make choices,
then choices make us. Choose an
inspiring destination, then create a set
of healthy habits to get you there.

JULY 4

*A good laugh and a long sleep are the
two best cures for anything.*
Irish Proverb

20__: _____

_____

_____

_____

20__: _____

_____

_____

_____

20__: _____

_____

_____

_____

REST – Rest rebuilds the mind, body,
and spirit. The best rest includes a
sanctuary of time set aside to rejuvenate
daily, weekly, and annually.

JULY 5

....

*Whether it is in your home, neighborhood, office,
or city make it your goal to push back the
jungle and recreate the garden.*
Des Cummings Jr., PhD

20__: _____

_____

_____

_____

20__: _____

_____

_____

_____

_____

20__: _____

_____

_____

_____

_____

E

ENVIRONMENT – All of your
senses—sight, smell, sound, touch, and
taste—influence your mood and your
health. So optimize your environment.

JULY 6

Exercise is medicine. Literally. Just like a pill, it reliably changes brain function by altering the activity of key brain chemicals and hormones.
Stephen S. Ilardi, PhD

20__: _____

_____

_____

_____

20__: _____

_____

_____

_____

20__: _____

_____

_____

_____

A **ACTIVITY** – Activity includes both mental and physical strengthening. A fit mind promotes a healthy body, and a healthy body promotes a fit mind.

JULY 7

. . . .

He longs to lead you, to show you hope and
a positive vision of your future.
Heather Neal

20__: _____

_____

_____

_____

20__: _____

_____

_____

_____

20__: _____

_____

_____

_____

TRUST – Trust in God can promote
better health. Faith, hope, and love
provide lasting peace and may help you
live a longer, happier life.

JULY 8

. . . .

Relationships are God's number one priority.
Des Cummings Jr., PhD

20__: _____

_____

_____

_____

20__: _____

_____

_____

_____

20__: _____

_____

_____

_____

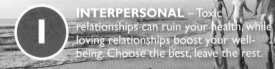

I **INTERPERSONAL** – Toxic
relationships can ruin your health, while
loving relationships boost your well-
being. Choose the best, leave the rest.

JULY 9

. . . .

*When it comes down to it, however, there is really only one
statistic that matters: I have been given one more day.*
Linda Nordyke Hambleton

20__: _____

_____

_____

_____

20__: _____

_____

_____

_____

20__: _____

_____

_____

_____

OUTLOOK – Attitude influences
outcome. Your outlook can impact the
progression of disease or the increase of
health. Choose to stay positive today.

JULY 10

Worship the Lord your God, and his blessing will be on your food and water. I will take away sickness from among you.
Exodus 23:25

20__: _____

_____

_____

_____

20__: _____

_____

_____

_____

20__: _____

_____

_____

_____

NUTRITION – Food is the fuel that drives your life. It can rev you up or slow you down. Evaluate your intake. Eat for energy. Eat for life!

JULY 11

You will succeed in whatever you choose to do,
and light will shine on the
road ahead of you.
Job 22:28

20___: _____

_____

_____

_____

20___: _____

_____

_____

_____

20___: _____

_____

_____

_____

CHOICE – First we make choices,
then choices make us. Choose an
inspiring destination, then create a set
of healthy habits to get you there.

JULY 12

You, Lord, give perfect peace even in turmoil to those who keep
their purpose firm and put their trust in you.
Isaiah 26:3 (Paraphrase)

20__: _____

_____

_____

_____

20__: _____

_____

_____

_____

20__: _____

_____

_____

_____

REST – Rest rebuilds the mind, body,
and spirit. The best rest includes a
sanctuary of time set aside to rejuvenate
daily, weekly, and annually.

JULY 13

. . . .

. . . my heart was refreshed by the reminder that beauty can be found in the most unlikely places and that we can beautifully and defiantly grow wherever we are planted.
Herdley Paolini, PhD

20__: _____

_____

_____

_____

20__: _____

_____

_____

_____

20__: _____

_____

_____

_____

E **ENVIRONMENT** – All of your senses—sight, smell, sound, touch, and taste—influence your mood and your health. So optimize your environment.

JULY 14

. . . .

*A man's health can be judged by which he
takes two at a time—pills or stairs.*
Joan Welsh

20__: _____

_____

_____

_____

20__: _____

_____

_____

_____

20__: _____

_____

_____

_____

ACTIVITY – Activity includes both
mental and physical strengthening. A fit
mind promotes a healthy body, and a
healthy body promotes a fit mind.

JULY 15

. . . .

Never will I leave you; never will I forsake you.
Hebrews 13:5 (NIV)

20__: _____

_____

_____

_____

20__: _____

_____

_____

_____

20__: _____

_____

_____

_____

TRUST – Trust in God can promote better health. Faith, hope, and love provide lasting peace and may help you live a longer, happier life.

JULY 16

. . . .

*We can choose the love, affirmation, and
openness we were designed for in an
environment of trust and security.*
Monica Reed, MD

20__: _____

_____

_____

_____

20__: _____

_____

_____

_____

20__: _____

_____

_____

_____

INTERPERSONAL – Toxic
relationships can ruin your health, while
loving relationships boost your well-
being. Choose the best, leave the rest.

JULY 17

. . . .

The greatest part of our happiness or misery
depends on our disposition and
not our circumstances.
George Washington

20__: _____

_____

_____

_____

20__: _____

_____

_____

_____

20__: _____

_____

_____

_____

OUTLOOK – Attitude influences
outcome. Your outlook can impact the
progression of disease or the increase of
health. Choose to stay positive today.

JULY 18

....

When you eat together with family,
you feast on love and laughter.
Des Cummings Jr., PhD

20__: _____

_____

_____

_____

20__: _____

_____

_____

_____

20__: _____

_____

_____

_____

NUTRITION – Food is the fuel that drives your life. It can rev you up or slow you down. Evaluate your intake. Eat for energy. Eat for life!

JULY 19

By the choices and acts of our lives,
we create the person that we are.
Kenneth Patton

20__: _____

_____

_____

_____

20__: _____

_____

_____

_____

20__: _____

_____

_____

_____

CHOICE – First we make choices, then choices make us. Choose an inspiring destination, then create a set of healthy habits to get you there.

JULY 20

. . . .

. . . to lie sometimes on the grass under trees on a summer's day,
listening to the murmur of the water, or watching the clouds
float across the sky, is by no means a waste of time.
John Lubbock

20__: _____

_____

_____

_____

20__: _____

_____

_____

_____

20__: _____

_____

_____

_____

REST – Rest rebuilds the mind, body, and spirit. The best rest includes a sanctuary of time set aside to rejuvenate daily, weekly, and annually.

JULY 21

*To sit in the shade on a fine day, and look upon verdure
is the most perfect refreshment.*
Jane Austen

20__: _____

_____

_____

_____

20__: _____

_____

_____

_____

20__: _____

_____

_____

_____

E

ENVIRONMENT –All of your
senses—sight, smell, sound, touch, and
taste—influence your mood and your
health. So optimize your environment.

JULY 22

. . . .

Ride a bicycle to visit a friend.
Des Cummings Jr., PhD

20__: _____

_____

_____

_____

20__: _____

_____

_____

_____

20__: _____

_____

_____

_____

ACTIVITY – Activity includes both mental and physical strengthening. A fit mind promotes a healthy body, and a healthy body promotes a fit mind.

JULY 23

. . . .

I believe in the sun even when it is not shining. I believe
in love even when I cannot feel it. I believe
in God even when he is silent.
Holocaust Prisoner

20__: _____

_____

_____

_____

20__: _____

_____

_____

_____

20__: _____

_____

_____

_____

TRUST – Trust in God can promote
better health. Faith, hope, and love
provide lasting peace and may help you
live a longer, happier life.

JULY 24

....

*The best security blanket a child can have
is parents who respect each other.*
Jane Blaustone

20__: _____

_____

_____

_____

20__: _____

_____

_____

_____

20__: _____

_____

_____

_____

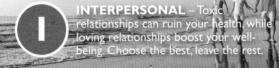

I

INTERPERSONAL – Toxic
relationships can ruin your health, while
loving relationships boost your well-
being. Choose the best, leave the rest.

JULY 25

. . . .

Live with hope and act with goodness.
Des Cummings Jr., PhD

20__: _____

_____

_____

_____

20__: _____

_____

_____

_____

20__: _____

_____

_____

_____

OUTLOOK – Attitude influences
outcome. Your outlook can impact the
progression of disease or the increase of
health. Choose to stay positive today.

JULY 26

....

It is my view that a vegetarian manner of living, by its purely
physical effect on human temperament, would most
beneficially influence the lot of mankind.
Albert Einstein

20__: _____

_____

_____

_____

20__: _____

_____

_____

_____

20__: _____

_____

_____

_____

NUTRITION – Food is the fuel that
drives your life. It can rev you up or slow
you down. Evaluate your intake. Eat for
energy. Eat for life!

JULY 27

*Our outlook often determines our choices,
and our choices impact our outlook.*
Kim Johnson

20__: _____

_____

_____

_____

20__: _____

_____

_____

_____

20__: _____

_____

_____

_____

CHOICE – First we make choices, then choices make us. Choose an inspiring destination, then create a set of healthy habits to get you there.

JULY 28

. . . .

Never discount the fact that resting is just as important as work.
Sometimes when I'm not motivated I use that time to
shut it down and take a rest day or two.
Lolo Jones

20__: _____

_____

_____

_____

20__: _____

_____

_____

_____

20__: _____

_____

_____

_____

REST – Rest rebuilds the mind, body, and spirit. The best rest includes a sanctuary of time set aside to rejuvenate daily, weekly, and annually.

JULY 29

In choosing colors ... follow nature's lead.
John Saladino

20__: _____

_____

_____

_____

20__: _____

_____

_____

_____

20__: _____

_____

_____

_____

E

ENVIRONMENT – All of your
senses—sight, smell, sound, touch, and
taste—influence your mood and your
health. So optimize your environment.

JULY 30

*When physically challenged through regular exercise,
the human body grows stronger and
healthier, and ages more slowly.*
Des Cummings Jr., PhD

20__: _____

_____

_____

_____

20__: _____

_____

_____

_____

20__: _____

_____

_____

_____

ACTIVITY – Activity includes both
mental and physical strengthening. A fit
mind promotes a healthy body, and a
healthy body promotes a fit mind.

JULY 31

. . . .

Call to me and I will answer you and show you great
and mighty things which you do not know.
Jeremiah 33:3 (NKJV)

20__: _____

_____

_____

_____

20__: _____

_____

_____

_____

20__: _____

_____

_____

_____

TRUST – Trust in God can promote
better health. Faith, hope, and love
provide lasting peace and may help you
live a longer, happier life.

AUGUST 1

. . . .

*A fundamental principle of dealing with
hardship is, "We're all in this together."*
Sandy Shugart, PhD

20__: _____

_____

_____

_____

20__: _____

_____

_____

_____

20__: _____

_____

_____

_____

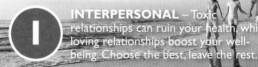

INTERPERSONAL – Toxic
relationships can ruin your health, while
loving relationships boost your well-
being. Choose the best, leave the rest.

AUGUST 2

A positive outlook can make the difference
between recovery and paralysis.
Des Cummings Jr., PhD

20__: _____

_____

_____

_____

20__: _____

_____

_____

_____

20__: _____

_____

_____

_____

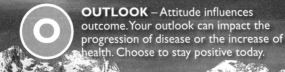

OUTLOOK – Attitude influences
outcome. Your outlook can impact the
progression of disease or the increase of
health. Choose to stay positive today.

AUGUST 3

He who distinguishes the true savor of his food can never be a glutton; he who does not cannot be otherwise.
Henry David Thoreau

20__: _____

_____

_____

_____

20__: _____

_____

_____

_____

20__: _____

_____

_____

_____

NUTRITION – Food is the fuel that drives your life. It can rev you up or slow you down. Evaluate your intake. Eat for energy. Eat for life!

AUGUST 4

. . . .

*What we call the secret of happiness is no more a secret
than our willingness to choose life.*
Leo Buscaglia

20__: _____

_____

_____

_____

20__: _____

_____

_____

_____

20__: _____

_____

_____

_____

CHOICE – First we make choices,
then choices make us. Choose an
inspiring destination, then create a set
of healthy habits to get you there.

AUGUST 5

. . . .

Then Jesus said, "Come to me, all of you who are weary and carry heavy burdens, and I will give you rest."
Matthew 11:28

20__: _____

_____

_____

_____

20__: _____

_____

_____

_____

20__: _____

_____

_____

_____

REST – Rest rebuilds the mind, body, and spirit. The best rest includes a sanctuary of time set aside to rejuvenate daily, weekly, and annually.

AUGUST 6

God enjoys beauty for beauty's sake.
Lynell LaMountain

20__: _____

_____

_____

_____

20__: _____

_____

_____

_____

20__: _____

_____

_____

_____

ENVIRONMENT – All of your senses—sight, smell, sound, touch, and taste—influence your mood and your health. So optimize your environment.

AUGUST 7

. . . .

Thirty minutes of physical exercise three times a week, and
fifteen minutes of laughter on a daily basis is strongly
recommended for the vascular system.
Michael Miller, MD

20__: _____

_____

_____

_____

20__: _____

_____

_____

_____

20__: _____

_____

_____

_____

ACTIVITY – Activity includes both
mental and physical strengthening. A fit
mind promotes a healthy body, and a
healthy body promotes a fit mind.

AUGUST 8

Very simply, prayer is relinquishing your greatest concerns to the Maker of the Universe.
Monica Reed, MD

20__: _____

_____

_____

_____

20__: _____

_____

_____

_____

20__: _____

_____

_____

_____

TRUST – Trust in God can promote better health. Faith, hope, and love provide lasting peace and may help you live a longer, happier life.

AUGUST 9

A greater love works through [my family] toward me.
Linda Nordyke Hambleton

20__: _____

_____

_____

_____

20__: _____

_____

_____

_____

20__: _____

_____

_____

_____

INTERPERSONAL – Toxic relationships can ruin your health, while loving relationships boost your well-being. Choose the best, leave the rest.

AUGUST 10

With the assurance of heaven's partnership, we can venture into uncharted territory in our abundant living journey.
Kim Johnson

20__: _____

_____

_____

_____

20__: _____

_____

_____

_____

20__: _____

_____

_____

_____

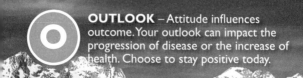

OUTLOOK – Attitude influences outcome. Your outlook can impact the progression of disease or the increase of health. Choose to stay positive today.

AUGUST 11

Try snacking on raw vegetables instead of crackers or chips.
Des Cummings Jr., PhD

20__: _____

_____

_____

_____

20__: _____

_____

_____

_____

20__: _____

_____

_____

_____

NUTRITION – Food is the fuel that drives your life. It can rev you up or slow you down. Evaluate your intake. Eat for energy. Eat for life!

AUGUST 12

....

We have to choose between what is right and what is easy.
J.K. Rowling

20__: _____

_____

_____

20__: _____

_____

_____

_____

20__: _____

_____

_____

_____

CHOICE – First we make choices, then choices make us. Choose an inspiring destination, then create a set of healthy habits to get you there.

AUGUST 13

. . . .

Sometimes you just need to take a nap and get over it.
Maura Stuard, age 8

20__: _____

_____

_____

_____

20__: _____

_____

_____

_____

20__: _____

_____

_____

_____

 REST – Rest rebuilds the mind, body, and spirit. The best rest includes a sanctuary of time set aside to rejuvenate daily, weekly, and annually.

AUGUST 14

. . . .

*Color does not add a pleasant quality
to design—it reinforces it.*
Pierre Bonnard

20__: _____

_____

_____

_____

20__: _____

_____

_____

_____

20__: _____

_____

_____

_____

ENVIRONMENT – All of your
senses—sight, smell, sound, touch, and
taste—influence your mood and your
health. So optimize your environment.

AUGUST 15

. . . .

The greatest gift we have is the gift of life … from our Creator.
We're given a body. Now you may not like it, but you can
maximize that body the best it can be …
Mike Ditka

20__: _____

_____

_____

_____

20__: _____

_____

_____

_____

20__: _____

_____

_____

_____

ACTIVITY – Activity includes both
mental and physical strengthening. A fit
mind promotes a healthy body, and a
healthy body promotes a fit mind.

AUGUST 16

*When did you last thank him for lavishing his free
and unconditional grace upon you?*
Dr. Dick Tibbits

20__: _____

_____

_____

_____

20__: _____

_____

_____

_____

20__: _____

_____

_____

_____

TRUST – Trust in God can promote
better health. Faith, hope, and love
provide lasting peace and may help you
live a longer, happier life.

AUGUST 17

. . . .

We are all a little weird, and when we find someone whose weirdness is compatible with ours, we join up with them and fall in a mutual weirdness and call it love.

Dr. Seuss

20__: _____

_____

_____

_____

20__: _____

_____

_____

_____

20__: _____

_____

_____

_____

INTERPERSONAL – Toxic relationships can ruin your health, while loving relationships boost your well-being. Choose the best, leave the rest.

AUGUST 18

....

*If you ask what the single most important key to
longevity, I would have to say it is avoiding
worry, stress, and tension.*
George Burns

20__: _____

_____

_____

_____

20__: _____

_____

_____

_____

20__: _____

_____

_____

_____

OUTLOOK – Attitude influences
outcome. Your outlook can impact the
progression of disease or the increase of
health. Choose to stay positive today.

AUGUST 19

To lengthen thy life, lessen thy meals.
Benjamin Franklin

20__: _____

_____

_____

_____

20__: _____

_____

_____

_____

20__: _____

_____

_____

_____

NUTRITION – Food is the fuel that drives your life. It can rev you up or slow you down. Evaluate your intake. Eat for energy. Eat for life!

AUGUST 20

The righteous choose their friends carefully, but the way of the wicked leads them astray.
Proverbs 12:26 (KJV)

20__: _____

_____

_____

_____

20__: _____

_____

_____

_____

20__: _____

_____

_____

_____

CHOICE – First we make choices, then choices make us. Choose an inspiring destination, then create a set of healthy habits to get you there.

AUGUST 21

. . . .

Take rest; a field that has rested
gives a beautiful crop.
Ovid

20__: _____

_____

_____

_____

20__: _____

_____

_____

_____

20__: _____

_____

_____

_____

REST – Rest rebuilds the mind, body, and spirit. The best rest includes a sanctuary of time set aside to rejuvenate daily, weekly, and annually.

AUGUST 22

*God writes the gospel not in the Bible alone,
but also on trees and in the flowers
and clouds and stars.*
Martin Luther

20__: _____

_____

_____

_____

20__: _____

_____

_____

_____

20__: _____

_____

_____

_____

E **ENVIRONMENT** – All of your senses—sight, smell, sound, touch, and taste—influence your mood and your health. So optimize your environment.

AUGUST 23

. . . .

If I can reconnect them to the positive things they remember
from when they were active, it's much easier
for them to get back into it again.
Rhonda Ringer, MD

20__: _____

_____

_____

_____

20__: _____

_____

_____

_____

20__: _____

_____

_____

_____

ACTIVITY – Activity includes both
mental and physical strengthening. A fit
mind promotes a healthy body, and a
healthy body promotes a fit mind.

AUGUST 24

. . . .

Besides that, trying to control things on my own isolates me from
the miracles of hope and joy that God can bring about
in the midst of pain and suffering.
Linda Nordyke Hambleton

20__: _____

_____

_____

_____

20__: _____

_____

_____

_____

20__: _____

_____

_____

_____

TRUST – Trust in God can promote
better health. Faith, hope, and love
provide lasting peace and may help you
live a longer, happier life.

AUGUST 25

. . . .

Let the wife make the husband glad to come home,
and let him make her sorry to see him leave.
Martin Luther

20__: _____

_____

_____

_____

20__: _____

_____

_____

_____

20__: _____

_____

_____

_____

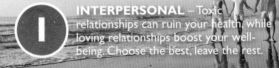

INTERPERSONAL – Toxic
relationships can ruin your health, while
loving relationships boost your well-
being. Choose the best, leave the rest.

AUGUST 26

....

*Pessimist: One who, when he has the
choice of two evils, chooses both.*
Oscar Wilde

20__: _____

_____

_____

_____

20__: _____

_____

_____

_____

20__: _____

_____

_____

_____

OUTLOOK – Attitude influences
outcome. Your outlook can impact the
progression of disease or the increase of
health. Choose to stay positive today.

AUGUST 27

To eat is a necessity, but to eat intelligently is an art.
La Rochefoucauld

20__: _____

_____

_____

_____

20__: _____

_____

_____

_____

20__: _____

_____

_____

_____

NUTRITION – Food is the fuel that drives your life. It can rev you up or slow you down. Evaluate your intake. Eat for energy. Eat for life!

AUGUST 28

. . . .

*When life isn't fair, we are left with two
choices—to blame or to forgive.*
Dr. Dick Tibbits

20__: _____

_____

_____

_____

20__: _____

_____

_____

_____

20__: _____

_____

_____

_____

CHOICE – First we make choices,
then choices make us. Choose an
inspiring destination, then create a set
of healthy habits to get you there.

AUGUST 29

. . . .

Once I knew what it was to rest upon the rock of
God's promises, and it was indeed a precious
resting place, but now I rest in His grace.
Hannah Whitall Smith

20__: _____

_____

_____

_____

20__: _____

_____

_____

_____

20__: _____

_____

_____

_____

REST – Rest rebuilds the mind, body,
and spirit. The best rest includes a
sanctuary of time set aside to rejuvenate
daily, weekly, and annually.

AUGUST 30

. . . .

Live in the sunshine, swim in the sea, drink the wild air. . . .
Ralph Waldo Emerson

20__: _____

_____

_____

_____

20__: _____

_____

_____

_____

20__: _____

_____

_____

_____

ENVIRONMENT – All of your senses—sight, smell, sound, touch, and taste—influence your mood and your health. So optimize your environment.

AUGUST 31

. . . .

Exercise is labor without weariness.
Samuel Johnson

20__: _____

_____

_____

_____

20__: _____

_____

_____

_____

20__: _____

_____

_____

_____

ACTIVITY – Activity includes both mental and physical strengthening. A fit mind promotes a healthy body, and a healthy body promotes a fit mind.

SEPTEMBER 1

When I am afraid, I will trust in you.
Psalm 56:3

20__: _____

_____

_____

20__: _____

_____

_____

20__: _____

_____

_____

_____

TRUST – Trust in God can promote better health. Faith, hope, and love provide lasting peace and may help you live a longer, happier life.

SEPTEMBER 2

*Be kinder than necessary because everyone you meet
is fighting some kind of battle.*
J.M. Barrie

20__: _____

_____

_____

_____

20__: _____

_____

_____

_____

20__: _____

_____

_____

_____

INTERPERSONAL – Toxic
relationships can ruin your health, while
loving relationships boost your well-
being. Choose the best, leave the rest.

SEPTEMBER 3

*I arise full of eagerness and energy, knowing well
what achievement lies ahead of me.*
Zane Grey

20__: _____

_____

_____

_____

20__: _____

_____

_____

_____

20__: _____

_____

_____

_____

OUTLOOK – Attitude influences
outcome. Your outlook can impact the
progression of disease or the increase of
health. Choose to stay positive today.

SEPTEMBER 4

*Man does not live on bread alone, but on every word
that comes from the mouth of God.*
Matthew 4:4

20__: _____

_____

_____

_____

20__: _____

_____

_____

_____

20__: _____

_____

_____

_____

NUTRITION – Food is the fuel that
drives your life. It can rev you up or slow
you down. Evaluate your intake. Eat for
energy. Eat for life!

SEPTEMBER 5

We cannot have full control over the number of years
we will live, but we can control the intensity
with which we will live them.
Des Cummings, Jr., PhD

20__: _____

_____

_____

_____

20__: _____

_____

_____

_____

20__: _____

_____

_____

_____

CHOICE – First we make choices,
then choices make us. Choose an
inspiring destination, then create a set
of healthy habits to get you there.

SEPTEMBER 6

Then I lay down and slept in peace and woke up safely,
for the Lord was watching over me.
Psalm 3:5 (TLB)

20__: _____

_____

_____

_____

20__: _____

_____

_____

_____

20__: _____

_____

_____

_____

REST – Rest rebuilds the mind, body, and spirit. The best rest includes a sanctuary of time set aside to rejuvenate daily, weekly, and annually.

SEPTEMBER 7

....

*Populations that are exposed to the greenest environments
have the lowest levels of health inequality
related to income deprivation.*
Richard Mitchell and Frank Popham

20___: _____

_____

_____

_____

20___: _____

_____

_____

_____

20___: _____

_____

_____

_____

E **ENVIRONMENT** – All of your
senses—sight, smell, sound, touch, and
taste—influence your mood and your
health. So optimize your environment.

SEPTEMBER 8

A body in motion tends to stay in motion,
and a body at rest tends to stay at rest.
Sir Isaac Newton

20__: _____

_____

_____

_____

20__: _____

_____

_____

_____

20__: _____

_____

_____

_____

ACTIVITY – Activity includes both mental and physical strengthening. A fit mind promotes a healthy body, and a healthy body promotes a fit mind.

SEPTEMBER 9

. . . .

As He has so many times, God and His peace met me there, again,
offering no real answers to my questions, but replacing the
anger with a joy that reached beyond my loss.
Linda Nordyke Hambleton

20___: _____

_____

_____

_____

20___: _____

_____

_____

_____

20___: _____

_____

_____

_____

TRUST – Trust in God can promote
better health. Faith, hope, and love
provide lasting peace and may help you
live a longer, happier life.

SEPTEMBER 10

*If there is any encouragement in Christ, any comfort in love . . .
any sympathy, complete my joy by having the same love,
being united, and agreeing with each other.*
Philippians 2:1-2 (CEB)

20__: _____

_____

_____

20__: _____

_____

_____

_____

20__: _____

_____

_____

_____

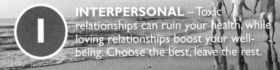

INTERPERSONAL – Toxic relationships can ruin your health, while loving relationships boost your well-being. Choose the best, leave the rest.

SEPTEMBER 11

*Determination, energy, and courage appear spontaneously
when we care deeply about something.*
Margret J. Wheatley

20__: _____

_____

_____

_____

20__: _____

_____

_____

_____

20__: _____

_____

_____

_____

OUTLOOK – Attitude influences
outcome. Your outlook can impact the
progression of disease or the increase of
health. Choose to stay positive today.

SEPTEMBER 12

*If it came from a plant, eat it; if it
was made in a plant, don't.*
Michael Pollan

20__: _____

_____

_____

_____

20__: _____

_____

_____

_____

20__: _____

_____

_____

_____

NUTRITION – Food is the fuel that
drives your life. It can rev you up or slow
you down. Evaluate your intake. Eat for
energy. Eat for life!

SEPTEMBER 13

Life is the way I decide it will be.
Des Cummings Jr., PhD

20__: _____

_____

_____

20__: _____

_____

_____

_____

20__: _____

_____

_____

_____

CHOICE – First we make choices, then choices make us. Choose an inspiring destination, then create a set of healthy habits to get you there.

SEPTEMBER 14

Rest when you're weary. Refresh and renew yourself,
your body, your mind, your spirit.
Then get back to work.
Ralph Marston

20__: _____

_____

_____

_____

20__: _____

_____

_____

_____

20__: _____

_____

_____

_____

REST – Rest rebuilds the mind, body,
and spirit. The best rest includes a
sanctuary of time set aside to rejuvenate
daily, weekly, and annually.

SEPTEMBER 15

*The whole world is charged with the glory of God
and I feel fire and music under my feet.*
Thomas Merton

20__: _____

_____

_____

_____

20__: _____

_____

_____

_____

20__: _____

_____

_____

_____

E

ENVIRONMENT – All of your
senses—sight, smell, sound, touch, and
taste—influence your mood and your
health. So optimize your environment.

SEPTEMBER 16

When it comes to eating right and exercising, there is no "I'll start tomorrow." Tomorrow is disease.
Terri Guillemets

20__: _____

_____

_____

_____

20__: _____

_____

_____

_____

20__: _____

_____

_____

_____

ACTIVITY – Activity includes both mental and physical strengthening. A fit mind promotes a healthy body, and a healthy body promotes a fit mind.

SEPTEMBER 17

When it comes to trials, we deposit ourselves into
God's safekeeping until that deposit
yields eternal dividends.
Charles Swindoll

20__: _____

_____

_____

_____

20__: _____

_____

_____

_____

20__: _____

_____

_____

_____

TRUST – Trust in God can promote
better health. Faith, hope, and love
provide lasting peace and may help you
live a longer, happier life.

SEPTEMBER 18

*Healthy relationships are gifts that keep on giving, producing
healing and wholeness for years to come.*
Des Cummings Jr., PhD

20__: _____

_____

_____

_____

20__: _____

_____

_____

_____

20__: _____

_____

_____

_____

I

INTERPERSONAL – Toxic
relationships can ruin your health, while
loving relationships boost your well-
being. Choose the best, leave the rest.

SEPTEMBER 19

*It is never too late to plant good thoughts and
good choices in the garden of the heart.*
Mark Laws

20__ : _____

_____

_____

_____

20__ : _____

_____

_____

_____

20__ : _____

_____

_____

_____

OUTLOOK – Attitude influences
outcome. Your outlook can impact the
progression of disease or the increase of
health. Choose to stay positive today.

SEPTEMBER 20

Blessed is the land…whose princes eat at a proper time—
for strength and not for drunkenness.
Ecclesiastes 10:17 (NIV)

20__: _____

_____

_____

_____

20__: _____

_____

_____

_____

20__: _____

_____

_____

_____

NUTRITION – Food is the fuel that drives your life. It can rev you up or slow you down. Evaluate your intake. Eat for energy. Eat for life!

SEPTEMBER 21

*Allow the world to live as it chooses, and allow
yourself to live as you choose.*
Richard Bach

20__ : _____

_____

_____

_____

20__ : _____

_____

_____

_____

20__ : _____

_____

_____

_____

CHOICE – First we make choices,
then choices make us. Choose an
inspiring destination, then create a set
of healthy habits to get you there.

SEPTEMBER 22

Finish each day before you begin the next, and interpose
a solid wall of sleep between the two.
Ralph Waldo Emerson

20__: _____

_____

_____

_____

20__: _____

_____

_____

_____

20__: _____

_____

_____

_____

REST – Rest rebuilds the mind, body, and spirit. The best rest includes a sanctuary of time set aside to rejuvenate daily, weekly, and annually.

SEPTEMBER 23

As the beauty of nature fills our senses daily, just imagine the surroundings of the first man and woman: pristine beauty, flora and fauna of every species, a full spectrum of colors, textures, oceans ... Monica Reed, MD

20__: _____

_____

_____

_____

20__: _____

_____

_____

_____

20__: _____

_____

_____

_____

ENVIRONMENT – All of your senses—sight, smell, sound, touch, and taste—influence your mood and your health. So optimize your environment.

SEPTEMBER 24

It's a lifestyle. Train like there's no finish line.
Unknown

20__: _____

_____

_____

_____

20__: _____

_____

_____

_____

20__: _____

_____

_____

_____

ACTIVITY – Activity includes both mental and physical strengthening. A fit mind promotes a healthy body, and a healthy body promotes a fit mind.

SEPTEMBER 25

....

Faith does not make things easy. It makes them possible.
Luke 1:37 (Paraphrase)

20__: _____

_____

_____

_____

20__: _____

_____

_____

_____

20__: _____

_____

_____

_____

TRUST – Trust in God can promote
better health. Faith, hope, and love
provide lasting peace and may help you
live a longer, happier life.

SEPTEMBER 26

The greatest gift is a portion of thyself.
Ralph Waldo Emerson

20__ : _____

_____

_____

_____

20__ : _____

_____

_____

_____

20__ : _____

_____

_____

_____

INTERPERSONAL – Toxic relationships can ruin your health, while loving relationships boost your well-being. Choose the best, leave the rest.

SEPTEMBER 27

. . . .

Why not go out on a limb? That's where the fruit is.
Mark Twain

20__ : _____

_____

_____

_____

20__ : _____

_____

_____

_____

20__ : _____

_____

_____

_____

OUTLOOK – Attitude influences outcome. Your outlook can impact the progression of disease or the increase of health. Choose to stay positive today.

SEPTEMBER 28

*Do not join those who drink too much wine or gorge themselves
on meat, for drunkards and gluttons become poor,
and drowsiness clothes them in rags.*
Proverbs 23:10-21 (NIV)

20__: _____

_____

_____

_____

20__: _____

_____

_____

_____

20__: _____

_____

_____

_____

NUTRITION – Food is the fuel that
drives your life. It can rev you up or slow
you down. Evaluate your intake. Eat for
energy. Eat for life!

SEPTEMBER 29

. . . .

If you limit your choice only to what seems possible or reasonable,
you disconnect yourself from what you truly want,
and all that is left is a compromise.
Robert Fritz

20__: _____

_____

_____

_____

20__: _____

_____

_____

_____

20__: _____

_____

_____

_____

CHOICE – First we make choices,
then choices make us. Choose an
inspiring destination, then create a set
of healthy habits to get you there.

SEPTEMBER 30

*Sometimes the most urgent and vital thing you can
possibly do is take a complete rest.*
Ashleigh Brilliant

20__: _____

_____

_____

_____

20__: _____

_____

_____

_____

20__: _____

_____

_____

_____

REST – Rest rebuilds the mind, body,
and spirit. The best rest includes a
sanctuary of time set aside to rejuvenate
daily, weekly, and annually.

OCTOBER 1

Rich colors are typical of a rich nature.
Van Day Truex

20__: _____

_____

_____

_____

20__: _____

_____

_____

_____

20__: _____

_____

_____

_____

ENVIRONMENT – All of your senses—sight, smell, sound, touch, and taste—influence your mood and your health. So optimize your environment.

OCTOBER 2

Commit to be fit.
Unknown

20__: _____

_____

_____

_____

20__: _____

_____

_____

_____

20__: _____

_____

_____

_____

ACTIVITY – Activity includes both mental and physical strengthening. A fit mind promotes a healthy body, and a healthy body promotes a fit mind.

OCTOBER 3

In inhalation and exhalation there is an energy and a lively divine spirit, since he, through his spirit supports the breath of life...
Michael Severetus

20__: _____

_____

_____

_____

20__: _____

_____

_____

_____

20__: _____

_____

_____

_____

TRUST – Trust in God can promote better health. Faith, hope, and love provide lasting peace and may help you live a longer, happier life.

OCTOBER 4

We must be our own before we can be another's.
Ralph Waldo Emerson

20__: _____

_____

_____

_____

20__: _____

_____

_____

_____

20__: _____

_____

_____

_____

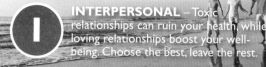

INTERPERSONAL – Toxic relationships can ruin your health, while loving relationships boost your well-being. Choose the best, leave the rest.

OCTOBER 5

. . . as a person moves out of denial and toward acceptance
of a condition, I don't think laughter is an
option; it's a requirement.
Linda Nordyke Hambleton

20__ : _____

_____

_____

_____

20__ : _____

_____

_____

_____

20__ : _____

_____

_____

_____

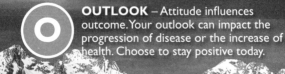

OUTLOOK – Attitude influences
outcome. Your outlook can impact the
progression of disease or the increase of
health. Choose to stay positive today.

OCTOBER 6

God gave you the sense of taste to enhance your life.
Des Cummings Jr., PhD

20__: _____

_____

_____

_____

20__: _____

_____

_____

_____

20__: _____

_____

_____

_____

NUTRITION – Food is the fuel that drives your life. It can rev you up or slow you down. Evaluate your intake. Eat for energy. Eat for life!

OCTOBER 7

*It's not hard to make decisions when you
know what your values are.*
Roy Disney

20__: _____

_____

_____

_____

20__: _____

_____

_____

_____

20__: _____

_____

_____

_____

CHOICE – First we make choices,
then choices make us. Choose an
inspiring destination, then create a set
of healthy habits to get you there.

OCTOBER 8

. . . .

The time to relax is when you don't have time for it.
Sydney J. Harris

20__: _____

_____

_____

_____

20__: _____

_____

_____

_____

20__: _____

_____

_____

_____

REST – Rest rebuilds the mind, body, and spirit. The best rest includes a sanctuary of time set aside to rejuvenate daily, weekly, and annually.

OCTOBER 9

*Tonight for dinner, actually sit at a table while not allowing any
outside distractions: No TV, no phone, no newspaper,
no mail, no work assignments.*
Des Cummings Jr., PhD

20__: _____

_____

_____

_____

20__: _____

_____

_____

_____

20__: _____

_____

_____

_____

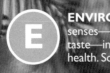

ENVIRONMENT – All of your
senses—sight, smell, sound, touch, and
taste—influence your mood and your
health. So optimize your environment.

OCTOBER 10

. . . .

Your body can do anything. It's just your
brain you have to convince.
Unknown

20__: _____

_____

_____

_____

20__: _____

_____

_____

_____

20__: _____

_____

_____

_____

ACTIVITY – Activity includes both
mental and physical strengthening. A fit
mind promotes a healthy body, and a
healthy body promotes a fit mind.

OCTOBER 11

What seems to us as bitter trials
are often blessings in disguise.
Oscar Wilde

20__: _____

_____

_____

_____

20__: _____

_____

_____

_____

20__: _____

_____

_____

_____

TRUST – Trust in God can promote
better health. Faith, hope, and love
provide lasting peace and may help you
live a longer, happier life.

OCTOBER 12

Today, take a few minutes to listen to someone's story.
You're likely to make a new friend.
Robyn Edgerton

20__: _____

_____

_____

_____

20__: _____

_____

_____

_____

20__: _____

_____

_____

_____

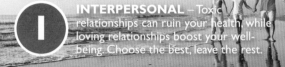

INTERPERSONAL – Toxic
relationships can ruin your health, while
loving relationships boost your well-
being. Choose the best, leave the rest.

OCTOBER 13

Whatever is true, whatever is noble, whatever is right, whatever is pure, whatever is lovely, whatever is admirable— if anything is excellent or praiseworthy—think about such things.
Philippians 4:8 (NIV)

20__: _____

_____

_____

_____

20__: _____

_____

_____

_____

20__: _____

_____

_____

_____

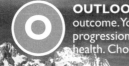

OUTLOOK – Attitude influences outcome. Your outlook can impact the progression of disease or the increase of health. Choose to stay positive today.

OCTOBER 14

. . . .

*Every time you eat or drink, you are either
feeding disease or fighting it.*
Heather Morgan

20__: _____

_____

_____

_____

20__: _____

_____

_____

_____

20__: _____

_____

_____

_____

NUTRITION – Food is the fuel that drives your life. It can rev you up or slow you down. Evaluate your intake. Eat for energy. Eat for life!

OCTOBER 15

*It's up to you today to start making healthy choices.
Not choices that are just healthy for your body,
but healthy for your mind.*
Steve Maraboli

20__: _____

_____

_____

_____

20__: _____

_____

_____

_____

20__: _____

_____

_____

_____

CHOICE – First we make choices,
then choices make us. Choose an
inspiring destination, then create a set
of healthy habits to get you there.

OCTOBER 16

*Rest time is not waste time. It is economy to gather fresh strength
. . . It is wisdom to take occasional furlough. In the long run, we
shall do more by sometimes doing less.*
Charles Spurgeon

20__: _____

_____

_____

_____

20__: _____

_____

_____

_____

20__: _____

_____

_____

_____

REST – Rest rebuilds the mind, body,
and spirit. The best rest includes a
sanctuary of time set aside to rejuvenate
daily, weekly, and annually.

OCTOBER 17

*The truly healthy environment is not
merely safe but stimulating.*
William H. Steward

20__: _____

_____

_____

_____

20__: _____

_____

_____

_____

20__: _____

_____

_____

_____

E

ENVIRONMENT – All of your
senses—sight, smell, sound, touch, and
taste—influence your mood and your
health. So optimize your environment.

OCTOBER 18

*Remember, physical activity is an indispensable key
to keeping those extra pounds at bay.*
Walt Larimore, MD

20__: _____

_____

_____

_____

20__: _____

_____

_____

_____

20__: _____

_____

_____

_____

ACTIVITY – Activity includes both
mental and physical strengthening. A fit
mind promotes a healthy body, and a
healthy body promotes a fit mind.

OCTOBER 19

God, who formed our being in the image of his own,
gives us stability and a sense of confidence that
we don't have to know it all or be it all.
Monica Reed, MD

20__: _____

_____

_____

_____

20__: _____

_____

_____

_____

20__: _____

_____

_____

_____

TRUST – Trust in God can promote
better health. Faith, hope, and love
provide lasting peace and may help you
live a longer, happier life.

OCTOBER 20

*Kindness is a currency that can cover a
multitude of interpersonal debts.*
George Alexiou

20__: _____

_____

_____

_____

20__: _____

_____

_____

_____

20__: _____

_____

_____

_____

INTERPERSONAL – Toxic
relationships can ruin your health, while
loving relationships boost your well-
being. Choose the best, leave the rest.

OCTOBER 21

Never lose an opportunity of seeing anything beautiful,
for beauty is God's handwriting.
Ralph Waldo Emerson

20__: _____

_____

_____

_____

20__: _____

_____

_____

_____

20__: _____

_____

_____

_____

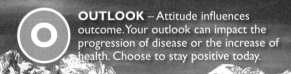

OUTLOOK – Attitude influences
outcome. Your outlook can impact the
progression of disease or the increase of
health. Choose to stay positive today.

OCTOBER 22

*In general, mankind, since the improvement of cookery,
eats twice as much as nature requires.*
Benjamin Franklin

20__: _____

_____

_____

_____

20__: _____

_____

_____

_____

20__: _____

_____

_____

_____

NUTRITION – Food is the fuel that
drives your life. It can rev you up or slow
you down. Evaluate your intake. Eat for
energy. Eat for life!

OCTOBER 23

. . . .

*Life is partly what we make it, and partly what it
is made by the friends we choose.*
Tennessee Williams

20__ : _____

_____

_____

_____

20__ : _____

_____

_____

_____

20__ : _____

_____

_____

_____

CHOICE – First we make choices,
then choices make us. Choose an
inspiring destination, then create a set
of healthy habits to get you there.

OCTOBER 24

....

Let a little water be brought, and then you may all
wash your feet and rest under this tree.
Genesis 18:4 (NKJV)

20__: _____

_____

_____

_____

20__: _____

_____

_____

_____

20__: _____

_____

_____

_____

REST – Rest rebuilds the mind, body,
and spirit. The best rest includes a
sanctuary of time set aside to rejuvenate
daily, weekly, and annually.

OCTOBER 25

One touch of nature makes the whole world kin.
William Shakespeare

20__: _____

_____

_____

_____

20__: _____

_____

_____

_____

20__: _____

_____

_____

_____

ENVIRONMENT – All of your senses—sight, smell, sound, touch, and taste—influence your mood and your health. So optimize your environment.

OCTOBER 26

*We can do nothing without the body, let us always take care
that it is in the best condition to sustain us.*
Socrates

20__: _____

_____

_____

_____

20__: _____

_____

_____

_____

20__: _____

_____

_____

_____

ACTIVITY – Activity includes both
mental and physical strengthening. A fit
mind promotes a healthy body, and a
healthy body promotes a fit mind.

OCTOBER 27

*Be anxious for nothing, but in everything by prayer
and supplication with thanksgiving let your
requests be made known to God.*
Philippians 4:6 (KJV)

20___: _____

_____

_____

_____

20___: _____

_____

_____

_____

20___: _____

_____

_____

_____

TRUST – Trust in God can promote
better health. Faith, hope, and love
provide lasting peace and may help you
live a longer, happier life.

OCTOBER 28

Love is infectious and the greatest healing energy.
Sai Baba

20__: _____

_____

_____

_____

20__: _____

_____

_____

_____

20__: _____

_____

_____

_____

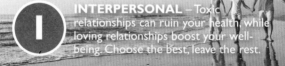

INTERPERSONAL – Toxic relationships can ruin your health, while loving relationships boost your well-being. Choose the best, leave the rest.

OCTOBER 29

．．．

*Write it on your heart that every day
is the best day in the year.*
Ralph Waldo Emerson

20__: _____

_____

_____

_____

20__: _____

_____

_____

_____

20__: _____

_____

_____

_____

OUTLOOK – Attitude influences
outcome. Your outlook can impact the
progression of disease or the increase of
health. Choose to stay positive today.

OCTOBER 30

I saw few die of hunger; of eating, a hundred thousand.
Benjamin Franklin

20__ : _____

_____

_____

_____

20__ : _____

_____

_____

_____

20__ : _____

_____

_____

_____

NUTRITION – Food is the fuel that drives your life. It can rev you up or slow you down. Evaluate your intake. Eat for energy. Eat for life!

OCTOBER 31

Choose your love. Love your choice.
Thomas S. Monson

20__: _____

_____

_____

_____

20__: _____

_____

_____

_____

20__: _____

_____

_____

_____

CHOICE – First we make choices, then choices make us. Choose an inspiring destination, then create a set of healthy habits to get you there.

NOVEMBER 1

Rest and be thankful.
William Wordsworth

20__: _____

_____

_____

_____

20__: _____

_____

_____

_____

20__: _____

_____

_____

_____

REST – Rest rebuilds the mind, body, and spirit. The best rest includes a sanctuary of time set aside to rejuvenate daily, weekly, and annually.

NOVEMBER 2

The mountains are calling and I must go.
John Muir

20__: _____

_____

_____

_____

20__: _____

_____

_____

_____

20__: _____

_____

_____

_____

E **ENVIRONMENT** – All of your senses—sight, smell, sound, touch, and taste—influence your mood and your health. So optimize your environment.

NOVEMBER 3

Exercise is good for your mind, body, and soul.
Susie Michelle Cortright

20__: _____

_____

_____

_____

20__: _____

_____

_____

_____

20__: _____

_____

_____

_____

ACTIVITY – Activity includes both mental and physical strengthening. A fit mind promotes a healthy body, and a healthy body promotes a fit mind.

NOVEMBER 4

*When we trust in God we are transformed from people of
fear to people of courage—and from people of
courage to people of purpose.*
Des Cummings Jr., PhD

20__: _____

_____

_____

_____

20__: _____

_____

_____

_____

20__: _____

_____

_____

_____

TRUST – Trust in God can promote
better health. Faith, hope, and love
provide lasting peace and may help you
live a longer, happier life.

NOVEMBER 5

. . . .

There is greatness in doing something you hate
for the sake of someone you love.
Shmuley Boteach

20___: _____

_____

_____

_____

20___: _____

_____

_____

_____

20___: _____

_____

_____

_____

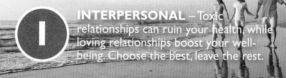

INTERPERSONAL – Toxic
relationships can ruin your health, while
loving relationships boost your well-
being. Choose the best, leave the rest.

NOVEMBER 6

. . . .

*Brick walls are there for a reason. They give
us a chance to show how badly
we want something.*
Randy Pausch

20__: _____

_____

_____

_____

20__: _____

_____

_____

_____

_____

20__: _____

_____

_____

_____

_____

OUTLOOK – Attitude influences
outcome. Your outlook can impact the
progression of disease or the increase of
health. Choose to stay positive today.

NOVEMBER 7

Here in America, we may talk healthy, but we eat tasty.
Sherri Flynt, MPH, RD, LD

20__: _____

_____

_____

_____

20__: _____

_____

_____

_____

20__: _____

_____

_____

_____

NUTRITION – Food is the fuel that drives your life. It can rev you up or slow you down. Evaluate your intake. Eat for energy. Eat for life!

NOVEMBER 8

You can't always control circumstances. However, you can always control your attitude.... Your options are to complain or to look ahead and figure out how to make the situation better.
Tony Dungy

20__: _____

_____

_____

_____

20__: _____

_____

_____

_____

20__: _____

_____

_____

_____

CHOICE – First we make choices, then choices make us. Choose an inspiring destination, then create a set of healthy habits to get you there.

NOVEMBER 9

A well-spent day brings happy sleep.
Leonardo Da Vinci

20__: _____

_____

_____

_____

20__: _____

_____

_____

_____

20__: _____

_____

_____

_____

REST – Rest rebuilds the mind, body, and spirit. The best rest includes a sanctuary of time set aside to rejuvenate daily, weekly, and annually.

NOVEMBER 10

*The human spirit needs places where nature has not
been rearranged by the hand of man.*
Author Unknown

20__: _____

_____

_____

_____

20__: _____

_____

_____

_____

20__: _____

_____

_____

_____

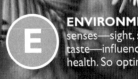

E **ENVIRONMENT** – All of your
senses—sight, smell, sound, touch, and
taste—influence your mood and your
health. So optimize your environment.

NOVEMBER 11

*If you don't do what's best for your body, you're the
one who comes up on the short end.*
Julius Erving

20__: _____

_____

_____

_____

20__: _____

_____

_____

_____

20__: _____

_____

_____

_____

ACTIVITY – Activity includes both
mental and physical strengthening. A fit
mind promotes a healthy body, and a
healthy body promotes a fit mind.

NOVEMBER 12

*But I trust in your unfailing love; my heart
rejoices in your salvation.*
Psalm 13:5

20__: _____

_____

_____

_____

20__: _____

_____

_____

_____

20__: _____

_____

_____

_____

TRUST – Trust in God can promote
better health. Faith, hope, and love
provide lasting peace and may help you
live a longer, happier life.

NOVEMBER 13

*One word frees us of all the weight and
pain of life: that word is love.*
Sophocles

20__: _____

_____

_____

_____

20__: _____

_____

_____

_____

20__: _____

_____

_____

_____

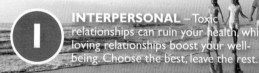

INTERPERSONAL – Toxic
relationships can ruin your health, while
loving relationships boost your well-
being. Choose the best, leave the rest.

NOVEMBER 14

....

Life ... It tends to respond to our outlook, to shape
itself to meet our expectation.
Richard DeVos

20__: _____

_____

_____

_____

20__: _____

_____

_____

_____

20__: _____

_____

_____

_____

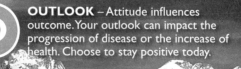

OUTLOOK – Attitude influences
outcome. Your outlook can impact the
progression of disease or the increase of
health. Choose to stay positive today.

NOVEMBER 15

*This is my invariable advice to people: learn how to cook.
Try new recipes, learn from your mistakes, be
fearless, and above all have fun!*
Julia Child

20__: _____

_____

_____

_____

20__: _____

_____

_____

_____

20__: _____

_____

_____

_____

NUTRITION – Food is the fuel that
drives your life. It can rev you up or slow
you down. Evaluate your intake. Eat for
energy. Eat for life!

NOVEMBER 16

The happiest people don't have the best of everything,
they just make the best of everything.
Unknown

20__: _____

_____

_____

_____

20__: _____

_____

_____

_____

20__: _____

_____

_____

_____

CHOICE – First we make choices, then choices make us. Choose an inspiring destination, then create a set of healthy habits to get you there.

NOVEMBER 17

*God says, "Come together and repair any cracks
in your relationships, reset the fractures
in your love for each other."*
Des Cummings Jr., PhD

20__: _____

_____

_____

_____

20__: _____

_____

_____

_____

20__: _____

_____

_____

_____

REST – Rest rebuilds the mind, body,
and spirit. The best rest includes a
sanctuary of time set aside to rejuvenate
daily, weekly, and annually.

NOVEMBER 18

We can never have enough of nature.
Henry David Thoreau

20__: _____

_____

_____

_____

20__: _____

_____

_____

_____

20__: _____

_____

_____

_____

ENVIRONMENT – All of your senses—sight, smell, sound, touch, and taste—influence your mood and your health. So optimize your environment.

NOVEMBER 19

. . . .

*Walking or running on the beach, at the park, or
around your neighborhood can be a welcome
change of pace from a treadmill.*
Monica Reed, MD

20__: _____

_____

_____

_____

20__: _____

_____

_____

_____

20__: _____

_____

_____

_____

ACTIVITY – Activity includes both
mental and physical strengthening. A fit
mind promotes a healthy body, and a
healthy body promotes a fit mind.

NOVEMBER 20

When the core of our being is threatened, that's when we find out that trust is not something you have; trust is something you do moment-by-moment.
Linda Nordyke Hambleton

20__: _____

_____

_____

_____

20__: _____

_____

_____

_____

20__: _____

_____

_____

_____

TRUST – Trust in God can promote better health. Faith, hope, and love provide lasting peace and may help you live a longer, happier life.

NOVEMBER 21

*When people think of you, do they get a warm feeling
knowing that you are caring, honest, trustworthy,
committed, and sincere?*
Theo Stewart

20__: _____

_____

_____

_____

20__: _____

_____

_____

_____

20__: _____

_____

_____

_____

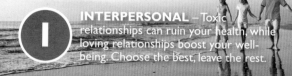

I

INTERPERSONAL – Toxic
relationships can ruin your health, while
loving relationships boost your well-
being. Choose the best, leave the rest.

NOVEMBER 22

....

Hope is not a way out but a way through.
Robert Frost

20__: _____

_____

_____

_____

20__: _____

_____

_____

_____

20__: _____

_____

_____

_____

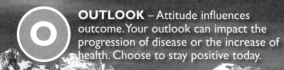

OUTLOOK – Attitude influences
outcome. Your outlook can impact the
progression of disease or the increase of
health. Choose to stay positive today.

NOVEMBER 23

....

*When it comes to healthy eating, people who know how
to cook and make ingredients taste good have a
distinct advantage over those who can't.*
Edward Ugel

20__: _____

_____

_____

_____

20__: _____

_____

_____

_____

20__: _____

_____

_____

_____

NUTRITION – Food is the fuel that
drives your life. It can rev you up or slow
you down. Evaluate your intake. Eat for
energy. Eat for life!

NOVEMBER 24

··

*The more you love your decisions, the less
you need others to love them.*
Unknown

20__: _____

_____

_____

_____

20__: _____

_____

_____

_____

20__: _____

_____

_____

_____

CHOICE – First we make choices,
then choices make us. Choose an
inspiring destination, then create a set
of healthy habits to get you there.

NOVEMBER 25

For fast-acting relief, try slowing down.
Lily Tomlin

20__: _____

_____

_____

_____

20__: _____

_____

_____

_____

20__: _____

_____

_____

_____

REST – Rest rebuilds the mind, body, and spirit. The best rest includes a sanctuary of time set aside to rejuvenate daily, weekly, and annually.

NOVEMBER 26

I thank you God for the leaping greenly spirits of trees, and for the blue dream of sky and for everything which is natural, which is infinite, which is yes.
e.e. cummings

20__: _____

_____

_____

_____

20__: _____

_____

_____

_____

20__: _____

_____

_____

_____

ENVIRONMENT – All of your senses—sight, smell, sound, touch, and taste—influence your mood and your health. So optimize your environment.

NOVEMBER 27

....

*Physical fitness can neither be achieved by wishful
thinking nor outright purchase.*
Joseph Pilates

20__: _____

_____

_____

_____

20__: _____

_____

_____

_____

20__: _____

_____

_____

_____

ACTIVITY – Activity includes both
mental and physical strengthening. A fit
mind promotes a healthy body, and a
healthy body promotes a fit mind.

NOVEMBER 28

Those who know your name trust in you, for you, Lord,
have never forsaken those who seek you.
Psalm 9:10 (NIV)

20___: _____

_____

_____

_____

20___: _____

_____

_____

_____

20___: _____

_____

_____

_____

TRUST – Trust in God can promote
better health. Faith, hope, and love
provide lasting peace and may help you
live a longer, happier life.

NOVEMBER 29

....

Without friends, it is very difficult for us
to get by, let alone thrive!
Tom Rath

20__: _____

_____

_____

_____

20__: _____

_____

_____

_____

20__: _____

_____

_____

_____

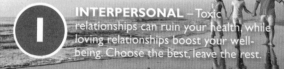

I

INTERPERSONAL – Toxic
relationships can ruin your health, while
loving relationships boost your well-
being. Choose the best, leave the rest.

NOVEMBER 30

*When you're curious, you find lots of
interesting things to do.*
Walt Disney

20__: _____

_____

_____

_____

20__: _____

_____

_____

_____

20__: _____

_____

_____

_____

OUTLOOK – Attitude influences
outcome. Your outlook can impact the
progression of disease or the increase of
health. Choose to stay positive today.

DECEMBER 1

....

*Cooking is at once child's play and adult joy. And
cooking done with care is an act of love.*
Craig Clairborne

20__: _____

_____

_____

_____

20__: _____

_____

_____

_____

20__: _____

_____

_____

_____

NUTRITION – Food is the fuel that
drives your life. It can rev you up or slow
you down. Evaluate your intake. Eat for
energy. Eat for life!

DECEMBER 2

We all find time to do what we really want to do.
William Feather

20__: _____

_____

_____

_____

20__: _____

_____

_____

_____

20__: _____

_____

_____

_____

CHOICE – First we make choices, then choices make us. Choose an inspiring destination, then create a set of healthy habits to get you there.

DECEMBER 3

20__: _____

_____

_____

_____

20__: _____

_____

_____

_____

20__: _____

_____

_____

_____

REST – Rest rebuilds the mind, body,
and spirit. The best rest includes a
sanctuary of time set aside to rejuvenate
daily, weekly, and annually.

DECEMBER 4

. . . .

Man's heart away from nature becomes hard.
Standing Bear

20__: _____

_____

_____

_____

20__: _____

_____

_____

_____

20__: _____

_____

_____

_____

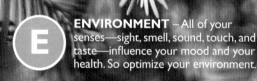

E **ENVIRONMENT** – All of your
senses—sight, smell, sound, touch, and
taste—influence your mood and your
health. So optimize your environment.

DECEMBER 5

The human body is made up of some four hundred muscles.... Unless they are used, they will deteriorate.
Eugene Lyman Fish

20__: _____

_____

_____

_____

20__: _____

_____

_____

_____

20__: _____

_____

_____

_____

ACTIVITY – Activity includes both mental and physical strengthening. A fit mind promotes a healthy body, and a healthy body promotes a fit mind.

DECEMBER 6

God changes caterpillars into butterflies, sand into pearls,
and coal into diamonds using time and pressure.
He's working on you, too.
Rick Warren

20__: _____

_____

_____

_____

20__: _____

_____

_____

_____

20__: _____

_____

_____

_____

TRUST – Trust in God can promote
better health. Faith, hope, and love
provide lasting peace and may help you
live a longer, happier life.

DECEMBER 7

Dining at home as a family can have a marked effect on reducing weight gain, as well as improving a family's physical, emotional, and relational health.
Sherri Flynt, MPH, RD, LD

20__: _____
_____
_____
_____

20__: _____
_____
_____
_____

20__: _____
_____
_____
_____

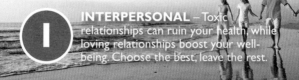

I **INTERPERSONAL** – Toxic relationships can ruin your health, while loving relationships boost your well-being. Choose the best, leave the rest.

DECEMBER 8

....

As you think, so shall you be.
Wayne W. Dyer

20__: _____

_____

_____

_____

20__: _____

_____

_____

_____

20__: _____

_____

_____

_____

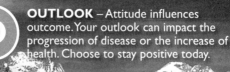

OUTLOOK – Attitude influences
outcome. Your outlook can impact the
progression of disease or the increase of
health. Choose to stay positive today.

DECEMBER 9

Eating may be a necessity, but enjoying the experience is not.
Des Cummings Jr., PhD

20__: _____

_____

_____

_____

20__: _____

_____

_____

_____

20__: _____

_____

_____

_____

NUTRITION – Food is the fuel that drives your life. It can rev you up or slow you down. Evaluate your intake. Eat for energy. Eat for life!

DECEMBER 10

Life is 10% what happens to you, and
90% how you react to it.
Charles Swindoll

20__: _____

_____

_____

_____

20__: _____

_____

_____

_____

20__: _____

_____

_____

_____

CHOICE – First we make choices, then choices make us. Choose an inspiring destination, then create a set of healthy habits to get you there.

DECEMBER 11

Sometimes the most important thing in a whole day is the
rest we take between two deep breaths.
Etty Hillesum

20__: _____

_____

_____

_____

20__: _____

_____

_____

_____

20__: _____

_____

_____

_____

REST – Rest rebuilds the mind, body,
and spirit. The best rest includes a
sanctuary of time set aside to rejuvenate
daily, weekly, and annually.

DECEMBER 12

....

Nature does not hurry, yet everything is accomplished.
Lao Tzu

20__: _____

_____

_____

_____

20__: _____

_____

_____

_____

20__: _____

_____

_____

_____

_____

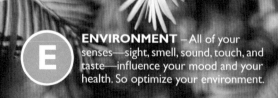

E **ENVIRONMENT** – All of your senses—sight, smell, sound, touch, and taste—influence your mood and your health. So optimize your environment.

DECEMBER 13

. . . .

Take the stairs instead of an elevator
at work whenever possible.
Des Cummings Jr., PhD

20__: _____

_____

_____

_____

20__: _____

_____

_____

_____

20__: _____

_____

_____

_____

ACTIVITY – Activity includes both mental and physical strengthening. A fit mind promotes a healthy body, and a healthy body promotes a fit mind.

DECEMBER 14

....

To believe in the supernatural is…simply to believe
that the supernatural is the greatest
reality here and now.
T. S. Eliot

20__: _____

_____

_____

_____

20__: _____

_____

_____

_____

20__: _____

_____

_____

_____

TRUST – Trust in God can promote
better health. Faith, hope, and love
provide lasting peace and may help you
live a longer, happier life.

DECEMBER 15

....

The best proof of love is trust.
Dr. Joyce Brothers

20__: _____

_____

_____

_____

20__: _____

_____

_____

_____

_____

20__: _____

_____

_____

_____

I

INTERPERSONAL – Toxic relationships can ruin your health, while loving relationships boost your well-being. Choose the best, leave the rest.

DECEMBER 16

We make a living by what we get.
We make a life by what we give.
Winston Churchill

20__: _____

_____

_____

_____

20__: _____

_____

_____

_____

20__: _____

_____

_____

_____

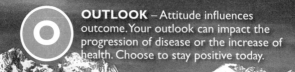

OUTLOOK – Attitude influences outcome. Your outlook can impact the progression of disease or the increase of health. Choose to stay positive today.

DECEMBER 17

....

My mom and Mario [Batali] taught me
the same lesson: Food is love.
Rachael Ray

20__: _____

_____

_____

_____

20__: _____

_____

_____

_____

20__: _____

_____

_____

_____

NUTRITION – Food is the fuel that
drives your life. It can rev you up or slow
you down. Evaluate your intake. Eat for
energy. Eat for life!

DECEMBER 18

. . . .

*If you're faced with a choice ... I hope you choose
the one that means the most to you.*
Jeffrey Steele

20__: _____

_____

_____

_____

20__: _____

_____

_____

_____

20__: _____

_____

_____

_____

_____

CHOICE – First we make choices,
then choices make us. Choose an
inspiring destination, then create a set
of healthy habits to get you there.

DECEMBER 19

Multitasking means you are living several experiences at the same time, under the illusion that more is better as you exchange peace for pace.
Des Cummings Jr., PhD

20__: _____

_____

_____

_____

20__: _____

_____

_____

_____

20__: _____

_____

_____

_____

REST – Rest rebuilds the mind, body, and spirit. The best rest includes a sanctuary of time set aside to rejuvenate daily, weekly, and annually.

DECEMBER 20

*How strange that nature does not knock,
and yet does not intrude!*
Emily Dickinson

20__: _____

_____

_____

_____

20__: _____

_____

_____

_____

20__: _____

_____

_____

_____

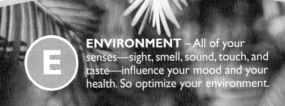

E **ENVIRONMENT** – All of your
senses—sight, smell, sound, touch, and
taste—influence your mood and your
health. So optimize your environment.

DECEMBER 21

....

*I just try to start my day with a good breakfast and
a quick walk, something simple that gets
the day off on the right foot.*
Natalie Coughlin

20__: _____

_____

_____

_____

20__: _____

_____

_____

_____

20__: _____

_____

_____

_____

ACTIVITY – Activity includes both
mental and physical strengthening. A fit
mind promotes a healthy body, and a
healthy body promotes a fit mind.

DECEMBER 22

*The truth is, you have captured God's
heart and won his affection.*
Todd Chobotar

20___: _____

_____

_____

_____

20___: _____

_____

_____

_____

20___: _____

_____

_____

_____

TRUST – Trust in God can promote
better health. Faith, hope, and love
provide lasting peace and may help you
live a longer, happier life.

DECEMBER 23

Alone we can do so little; together we can do so much.
Helen Keller

20__: _____

_____

_____

_____

20__: _____

_____

_____

_____

20__: _____

_____

_____

_____

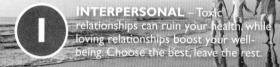

I **INTERPERSONAL** – Toxic relationships can ruin your health, while loving relationships boost your well-being. Choose the best, leave the rest.

DECEMBER 24

Life has always been a battle. Life has always been worth it.
Linda Nordyke Hambleton

20__: _____

_____

_____

_____

20__: _____

_____

_____

_____

20__: _____

_____

_____

_____

OUTLOOK – Attitude influences outcome. Your outlook can impact the progression of disease or the increase of health. Choose to stay positive today.

DECEMBER 25

. . . .

The more you eat, the less flavor;
the less you eat, the more flavor.
Proverb

20__: _____

_____

_____

_____

20__: _____

_____

_____

_____

20__: _____

_____

_____

_____

NUTRITION – Food is the fuel that drives your life. It can rev you up or slow you down. Evaluate your intake. Eat for energy. Eat for life!

DECEMBER 26

Today, I will be the best version of me.
Unknown

20__: _____

_____

_____

_____

20__: _____

_____

_____

_____

20__: _____

_____

_____

_____

CHOICE – First we make choices, then choices make us. Choose an inspiring destination, then create a set of healthy habits to get you there.

DECEMBER 27

He that can take rest is greater than he that can take cities.
Benjamin Franklin

20__: _____

_____

_____

_____

20__: _____

_____

_____

_____

20__: _____

_____

_____

_____

REST – Rest rebuilds the mind, body, and spirit. The best rest includes a sanctuary of time set aside to rejuvenate daily, weekly, and annually.

DECEMBER 28

Nature brings healing to the body, mind, and spirit.
Des Cummings Jr., PhD

20__: _____

_____

_____

_____

20__: _____

_____

_____

_____

20__: _____

_____

_____

_____

ENVIRONMENT – All of your senses—sight, smell, sound, touch, and taste—influence your mood and your health. So optimize your environment.

DECEMBER 29

Lack of activity destroys the good condition of every human being, while movement and methodical exercise save and preserve it.
Plato

20__: _____

_____

_____

_____

20__: _____

_____

_____

_____

20__: _____

_____

_____

_____

ACTIVITY – Activity includes both mental and physical strengthening. A fit mind promotes a healthy body, and a healthy body promotes a fit mind.

DECEMBER 30

....

*The only One who can truly satisfy the human
heart is the One who made it.*
Unknown

20__: _____

_____

_____

_____

20__: _____

_____

_____

_____

20__: _____

_____

_____

_____

TRUST – Trust in God can promote
better health. Faith, hope, and love
provide lasting peace and may help you
live a longer, happier life.

DECEMBER 31

When we're isolated, alone and disconnected, we suffer.
Monica Reed, MD

20__: _____
_____
_____
_____

20__: _____
_____
_____
_____

20__: _____
_____
_____
_____

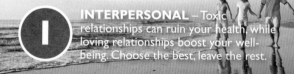

I

INTERPERSONAL – Toxic relationships can ruin your health, while loving relationships boost your well-being. Choose the best, leave the rest.

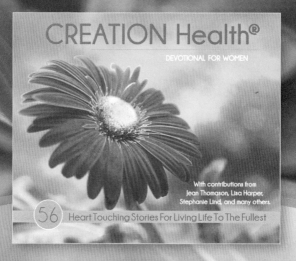

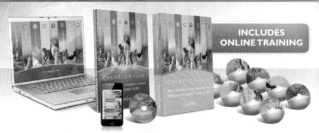
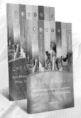

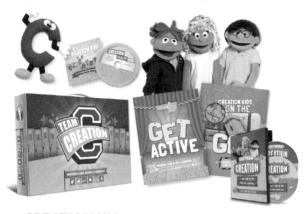

CREATION Kids

CREATION Health Kids can make a big difference in homes, schools, and congregations. Lead kids in your community to healthier, happier living.

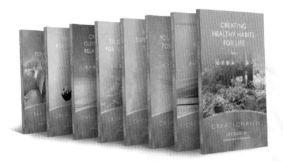

Life Guide Series

These guides include questions designed to help individuals or small groups study the depths of every principle and learn strategies for integrating them into everyday life.

CREATION HEALTH

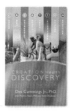

CREATION Health Discovery
(Softcover)

CREATION Health Discovery takes the 8 essential principles of CREATION Health and melds them together to form the blueprint for the health we yearn for and the life we are intended to live.

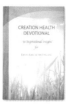

CREATION Health Devotional
(English) (Hardcover)

Devocionales De Salud CREACIÓN
(Spanish) (Softcover)

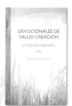

Stories change lives. Stories can inspire health and healing. In this devotional you will discover stories about experiencing God's grace in the tough times, God's delight in triumphant times, and God's presence in peaceful times. Based on the eight timeless principles of wellness: Choice, Rest, Environment, Activity, Trust, Interpersonal relationships, Outlook, Nutrition.

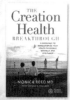

CREATION Health Breakthrough
(Hardcover)

Blending science and lifestyle recommendations, Monica Reed, MD, prescribes eight essentials that will help reverse harmful health habits and prevent disease. Discover how intentional choices, rest, environment, activity, trust, relationships, outlook, and nutrition can put a person on the road to wellness. Features a three-day total body rejuvenation therapy and four-phase life transformation plan.

QUICK REFERENCE GUIDE

....

Need some ideas for what to write about?

- ☐ Sum up your day in one sentence.

- ☐ Jot down something for which you are grateful.

- ☐ Create a short prayer.

- ☐ How did you live out your life purpose today?

- ☐ Write about something that made you smile.

- ☐ Copy a favorite quote you came across.

- ☐ Who were you with today and what did you do together?

- ☐ Something that made you sad or reflective today.

- ☐ Make note of medical treatment.

- ☐ Compose a haiku or short poem.

- ☐ What great idea did you have today?